My RA: A 50 Year Journey *and what I have learnt on the way*

By

Jasmine Jenkins

Shield Crest

ISBN: 978-1-917525-57-2

MMXXV

A CIP catalogue record for this book
is available from the British Library.

Published by
ShieldCrest Publishing,
Boston, Lincolnshire,
PE20 3BT England
Tel: +44 (0) 333 8000 890
www.shieldcrest.co.uk

Acknowledgements

Firstly, I want to say a big thank you to all the people who read and reviewed my manuscript and gave me the confidence to seek publication; Anne, Ailsa, Carolyn, Jan, Keith, Pam and Sharon thank you all for your help. A special mention for Ailsa. Thank you for finding the time in your busy schedule as NRAS founder and Patient Champion to read through my book and write a foreward for me. It reassured me that it all made sense! Carolyn, you were an amazing editor and proof reader so a special thank you for doing that for me. And of course I must mention my Keith; what would I do without your support in all my endeavours? You have shared my life for all of the fifty years with RA and I maybe wasn't what you bargained for! I appreciate all that you have done to support me. Lastly, I would like to thank my local SGI Buddhist group for the inspiration to write this book.

Contents

About the Author

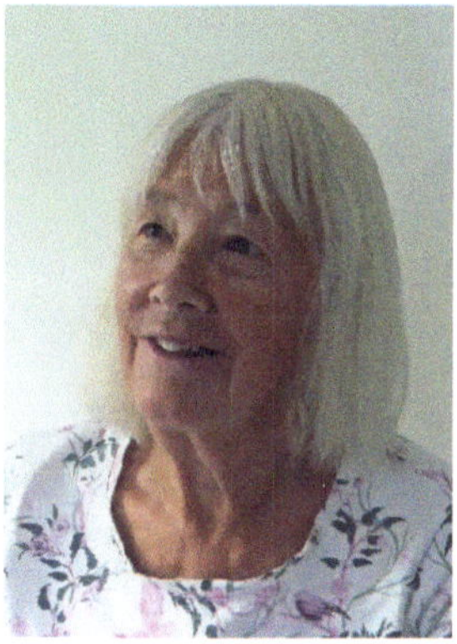

At the age of 22, Jasmine Jenkins started to experience pain, swelling and stiffness in her fingers, wrists and toes. For many years she had no idea why this was happening. At 32 she was eventually diagnosed with Rheumatoid Arthritis. At 40, she decided to train as an occupational therapist to help others with chronic conditions and disabilities.

In 2005 the first edition of her self-help book on RA was published. Now, after living with RA for over 50 years, she has decided it's time for a new book. Jasmine continues her involvement with the National Rheumatoid Arthritis Society[1], She still enjoys many of the things that she loves, including travelling with Keith in their beloved but ancient caravan.

---

[1] 50 % of the royalties from this book will be donated to NRAS

Foreword

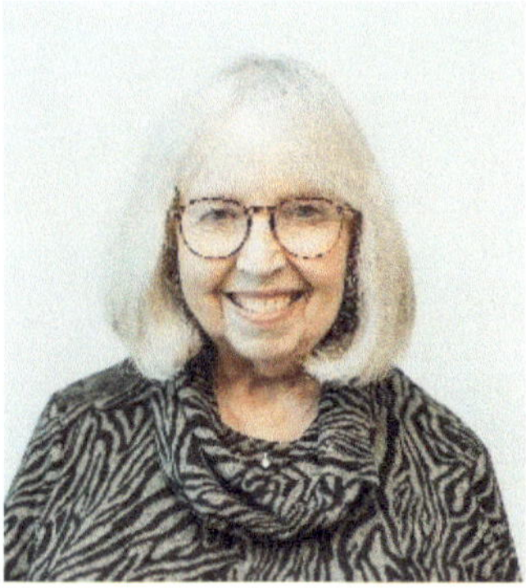

By Ailsa Bosworth, MBE

Founder and National Patient Champion

The National Rheumatoid Arthritis Society, NRAS

It is a pleasure and an honour to write the foreword for Jasmine's new book, 'My RA: A 50 Year Journey'. My journey is almost as long at some 46 years, I have to say that I relived many moments in my own life reading this. So many situations resonated, right through from diagnosis as a young working woman, having a young family (although I only had 1 daughter) and all the struggles that dealing with small people brings when you have really painful hands and wrists and getting established in a career that you are passionate about.

Some moments in the book brought a smile to my face and some a tear. For example, the danger of getting locked in the loo and unable to get out! My husband bought me a very natty little pair of pliers to deal with just such a situation which I forgot were in my handbag, and thus found them confiscated going through Heathrow 😊

If you know nothing about RA, as is so eloquently described

in this book, you are oblivious to the pain, fatigue and other debilitating symptoms that people with RA experience which are usually invisible, and this can sometimes appear uncaring and even callous. It's easy to get upset when you experience an able-bodied young person parking in a disabled slot for example, who then shouts at you when you ask them to move. Or, when an employer treats you in a way which threatens your ability to keep your job. These types of situations mean that to survive well, you really do need to develop resilience and coping strategies as well as learn as much as you can about your disease and how to self-manage with the right support, as so well argued here.

Gradually losing your ability to do things that you love is an ongoing grieving process that you also have to learn to come to terms with. Like Jasmine, I have lots of foot and ankle problems having had numerous major surgeries on both feet and ankles, and I too find walking on slopes and uneven ground really difficult and so miss being able to go for a long walk. Maintaining whatever exercise you can, is so important and there is much good advice within these pages relating to joint movement as well as joint protection techniques.

Many people will find the Appendix with all the many excellent top tips on how to do things incredibly useful. Jasmine's knowledge as an Occupational Therapist (OT) for many years has really highlighted the enormous value that OT's and the wider members of the rheumatology multi-disciplinary team bring. However, we know that the current NHS Workforce shortages in rheumatology mean that sadly not everyone has access to a specialist rheumatology OT. The good news, as emphasised by Jasmine throughout her book, is that for those diagnosed since the advent of biologics circa 2000, their journey will be very different to ours, and that really is to be celebrated. Much exciting research is being done and the fight against RA continues!

Introduction

During the last five years I have increasingly spent more and more time and energy getting to medical appointments, chasing them up, struggling with pain and trying my best to remain independent. My life has, at times, become a bit of a battle, where I am fighting to keep on doing the things that I love and trying to be as active as I can, every day. Sometimes I ask myself the question 'why have I had to cope with all these difficulties for so long', almost all of my adult life in fact, as my RA started when I was only 22.

In the last four years I have been practising and studying SGI Buddhism and one of the very wonderful ideas from this practise is learning to be resilient; taking on the difficult challenges that we all have in our lives and transforming them into something good. "Turning poison into medicine" is what we call this. From this principal I had the realisation that I could use all my experience of living with RA to write a second book. This time around I would write about the challenges I've faced during each decade, discuss my successes and my frustrations and also talk about the things that I have learnt about managing my RA along the way. Even better, I could also highlight the many things that have improved during these 50 years for people being diagnosed with RA now and how much brighter their future is.

I wrote my previous book, a self-help guide for people with RA twenty years ago. I was looking for ideas for managing my condition and I could barely find any helpful books at all. Being an Occupational Therapist [OT] I realised that I had the experience and a unique perspective to write a self-help book. I had never intended to write a book then and I certainly was not intending to write another one! My last book had three editions and is still available but there have been some very positive changes since then for people diagnosed with RA, so, I definitely feel that it's the right time for a new book with a different format and focus that will still be helpful for people with RA.

To make a start I decided to write a paragraph a day on Facebook for RA Awareness week, a blog about the challenges I have faced in each decade of my adult life; a decade a day for five days. After this I thought I would write a diary for the month of October to remind myself of my daily challenges and successes. This would allow me to see whether writing a book would be useful. As I started writing the diary, the ideas for the book took shape and it has been cathartic for me to reminisce and also quite exciting thinking about all the positive changes that are now improving the lives of people with RA. I really hope you will enjoy this journey through my 50 years of living with RA.

My October Diary.

Oct 1st

Today we went to visit our daughter who lives on a very steep hill. The first obstacle was parking. Our daughter has a permit, but this of course does not necessarily guarantee us a space anywhere near her house! Sometimes Keith, my husband, has to drop me and park elsewhere. Also, the scooter cannot go into the flat due to the stairs so if we want to go out somewhere then the scooter has to be collected from wherever the parking is and then returned!! I have no ankle movement so walking the very short distance up or down this steep hill from the car is very difficult and scary, so I often need to hang on to Keith.

The next obstacle is the steep staircase with a turn at the top, although we have had rails installed and these really help. There is a turn at the top that is tricky and again quite scary for me. I never used to be a person who had any fear, so my RA and disabilities along with getting older have made me a lot more careful, especially in the last few years, and I can never be spontaneous. We visited a pub which was quite spacious so the scooter could be stored without navigating around peoples' seats, but it was fortunate I could walk into the toilet as there was no wheelchair space or room to transfer due to all the clutter in the way. Many toilets are used for storage or have bins where the space for wheelchairs is supposed to be. At least I could lock the toilet door though without fear of becoming trapped inside and that's not always the case for me!

Of course, roads and pavements are very hazardous for mobility scooters as you never know where a drop kerb will be or where there are obstacles on the pavement which you cannot get past. I would never go out on the mobility scooter alone unless in my local area and even then, things can change each day.

Oct 2nd

Today we spent time with our youngest grandchildren aged 2 and 4 We went to the playground, which they love, but my role has gradually reduced since my oldest grandson was born. He's 14 now. I can just about push a swing, but I cannot lift the little ones onto it. I have to lean against poles if there are no seats and if I have to walk more than five minutes at a time then we need to take the mobility scooter. I would love to be with them helping them onto the slides and climbing frames, but I just don't have the ability to do this now. I have always loved being involved but I am now reduced to being a bystander and it makes me feel like a voyeur at times. Of course, I cannot take them out on my own anymore either. At my house it's a bit easier. I can do activities at a table and get drinks and food, but little children love playing on the floor and 2 year olds need diversions every few minutes and they are always on the move. Also, I get stuck with opening things or building Lego or reaching and lifting things out of cupboards. Still, as I can't pick things up without a lot of difficulty, that's one job I don't need to do! I have to take care not to fall over things though!

Oct 3rd

Today I went to the zoo. I have a membership so I can just drive in for an hour or two and park where I like on the route. I have always loved animals and nature, and the walking does me good even if it's just a few minutes here and there. It gives me the motivation to walk a bit even with pain. I can park close to some of the animals and the toilets too.

Today in the evening I went to my singing group which I also love. My blue badge allows me close parking and even now, with a lot of pain and many limitations I have managed to go nearly every week. We do dance moves with some of our songs which used to be great for exercise but recently since the sciatica and back pain I sit some of the time and sing and do as many moves as I am able. It's really great fun though and I always say any exercise is better than none!

Oct 4th

Today I went to assess a potential reader in the local library as part of my volunteer coordinator role for Read Easy, a charity who coach adults to learn to read. There were no close blue badge spaces, so I had to park in the closest car park. I always carry minimal items in a rucksack on my shoulder as my reduced hand function and damaged joints mean that I cannot carry a bag. It's only about 150-200 metres but I have to perch on a seat or wall or otherwise lean on a fence halfway. Once in the library, our place is booked ahead so it's plain sailing once I'm there. I do wish there was a lot more seats in town centres. It would really help people with limited mobility and maybe more people would go to town and get more exercise if they had more places to rest.

Oct 5th

Today I had to go to town for the GP and then repark as I wanted to get a birthday card. The GP went well as I could use a blue badge space outside but there are only 2 blue badge spaces and often there's no parking in the car park at all. If I use non blue badge spaces, then I can't be sure that I will be able to squeeze myself into the car when I return as I need to open the door wide to get in! The spaces seem to get smaller and smaller, but I guess the cars are getting bigger and bigger, so I often have to park on a nearby double yellow line! Next, I drove further in and parked near the Post Office and the shop that I needed. I made it to the first one by sitting on a seat halfway, and then I was lucky as there was no queue in the Post Office, but I still had to walk 70 metres further to the card shop. By the time I found a card and paid I was in agony with pain and there were no seats, so I staggered to a nearby wall to recover. Another 100 metres and I was back in the car and so relieved. This is why I rarely go to a shop and why blue badge parking is so essential. The internet is a godsend for me too for most of my shopping and so are contactless cards which mean I don't have to spend ages tipping coins out of my purse with a queue of annoyed and frustrated people behind me!

Oct 6th

Hurray! Today I at last received clarification that I could have my elbow replacement operation. I have been waiting over two years for this. I have been losing muscle strength in my right arm due to the nerve pain shooting right down my arm as the ulna nerve became trapped under the joint. Hopefully this was the last hurdle. I had to have scans on my cervical spine to ensure it was stable enough for the surgery to go ahead. Now just the pre-op to go, however, it will probably be a few months yet.

My shopping delivery came this morning. This is a variable experience depending on who brings it in. I have ordered online since 2004 after a head on collision which left my husband Keith and I both in wheelchairs for a few months! It was a life saver then and also during covid except that so many people ordered at that time that I ended up sitting up until 12 00 when new delivery times became available! Even this was tricky with the timings. During covid it was all dropped on the step in a plastic crate and had to be transferred into a washing basket or two and then lifted in. Since then, some delivery drivers are still reluctant to come in although most do eventually. I have to make sure I'm not alone as I can't lift it in due to my very limited hand function and I can only get things out one at a time from the right height! Some drivers bring the crate straight in and help to take the shopping out while others just stand around or wait outside. Of course, it's much quicker for all of us if they do help us. It would be easier for us if all the drivers were aware that we would need help but there are different drivers most of the time and they all have to rush to get all the deliveries done and some are definitely more understanding than others.

Oct 7th

Visited my sister for the day. It's 40 miles each way so I am so glad I have my electric auto corsa courtesy of Motability! It is so easy to drive that I can feel 'normal' when I'm driving. The controls are easy, there's auto lights, the steering is light, the seat is comfy and there's a camera for reversing and parking. Best of all I can charge it up on my driveway. For years I have had to ask Keith to fill it up with petrol. I am so grateful to Motability for this electric car. Driving gives me freedom even when my walking is so limited. Even better the charging unit was put in for free!

Later on, I was making a list and packing for our imminent caravan trip. I can manage the case with a few sit-downs every few minutes and I usually take everything out to the caravan too. Keith does the lifting and hooking up. Of course, nowadays my mobility scooter always comes with me

Oct 8th

Drove to Knaresborough caravan site stopping for coffee on route. Of course, there's no blue badge close parking for caravans, but I managed to find a bench fairly close to the caravan and Keith collected the coffees. Once we arrived on the site my Keith sorted everything; He put the caravan legs down, plugged in the electric and connected the calorgaz and then collected the water. I used to help him with some of this but now I just have to sit in the car and wait patiently. I can't even reach the stuff in the back of the cupboards now to get the cuppa ready as I seem to be shrinking! Sometimes it's very frustrating being me. At least we still get to go though and I'm great at researching and planning which Keith would never get around to doing!

We had a quick look around the centre of the town, planning where I could take the scooter along the river without meeting steps! The view down to the gorge and viaduct was wonderful. We were up on the hill with the castle ruins, I was racing around the hill on my scooter!

Oct 9th

Visit to Shipton's cave. [Knaresborough] As usual I phoned ahead about accessibility. Many places want you to book online these days, but you really don't want to be booking expensive tickets if you cannot manage to see or experience very much. The person I spoke to was very helpful and told us to park within the grounds and gave us directions. She also reduced our entry price. We walked along the river with stunning views but the cave, well and falls were only reached by four lots of very steep steps so unfortunately it was not possible for me to get to them. I had a hot chocolate, some delicious cake and a chat with the helpful assistant who carried my chocolate. [You can't carry and steer the mobility scooter!] Keith took some photos of the attractions I missed! It can be quite frustrating at times, but I am used to it by now. I always think it's better to see what you can rather than miss everything and sometimes there are bonuses like having more time to read and digest information, observing extra nature like birds, butterflies and plants, taking more creative photos or just enjoying a chat! The view down to the viaduct was spectacular and I saw it from the top as well as both sides of the river.

Oct 10th

We visited Fountain Abbey [NT] An ancient abbey with extensive grounds and water gardens. It is on a very large scale so the distance from the Abbey ruins to the gigantic water gardens, cafe and toilets is a fair way and with the scooter we have to decide whether the scooter has enough charge to make it all around the site and back! The distance the scooter battery can manage should be 8 miles, but we wouldn't trust it past 6. If it's uphill or there is bumpy, rough ground it will use up more charge. In the past we have tried to visit two places without a recharge in the middle and found ourselves with one light remaining indicating that it will stop fairly soon! It's not an exact science so we don't know exactly how long we have left. Once Keith had to push it while I walked about 70 metres and then I got back on, and we alternated like that until the scooter just made it back into the caravan park! We are very careful now.

Oct 11th

We drove to another site and then decided to drive to Haworth, the home of the Bronte sisters. It was cold and misty as you might expect as it was the Yorkshire moors and the setting for Wuthering Heights. It was very cold for my hands on the mobility scooter. We were walking along a street near the museum when suddenly we arrived at Haworth village. It was very surprising because everything changed so quickly, and suddenly, it looked as if we were in the middle of a movie set! We were on a very steep and cobbled street which was very tricky to manoeuvre down on a scooter. It was full of cafes, shops, pubs and artisan shops which did feel a bit touristy and contrived. We didn't attempt the bottom half of the street which dropped steeply down, the cobbles made it impossible for me anyway, but the view down was wonderful and we took a couple of photos. We then went to warm up with a coffee in an excellent delicatessen which doubled up as a cafe and an evening restaurant.

Oct 12th

Today we visited Halifax Piece Hall. It is an amazing refurbishment of the ancient Cloth Hall. It is now used for events in the large central area with shops on the upper and lower levels and of course cafes and restaurants too. There was also a very interesting visitor centre telling the history with lots of photos. Later on when we were having a coffee I rode off on my scooter to access the toilets. This is when things became difficult. I had to go through double doors which had no automatic option and did not stay open even if you opened them. Luckily someone saw me and let me through. I then had to go down two floors in the lift, but when the lift arrived, the corridor outside was really narrow so I had to get off and manually drag the scooter round. On the way back I tried reversing along the corridor so that I could turn into the lift. It was easier but still tight. Going back up again I had to do about a 21 point turn to access the ground floor corridor! I did explain this all to the visitor centre receptionist. It was clearly not designed with people in wheelchairs or mobility scooters in mind.

Oct 13th

Today we had to drive home. Not much to report disability wise except that we were pleasantly surprised to see disabled drop off and some caravan spaces very near the entry to the services! This was most unusual and especially appreciated as it was bucketing down with rain. We normally tend to have a break every 90 minutes to help with counteracting my RA stiffness. I needed to get out stretch and walk a bit. Since I went onto Baricitinib, my latest RA medication, I don't get as stiff which makes travelling easier.

Oct 14th

A day of putting things away and doing washing so I was alternating jobs that needed sitting, standing and walking. Over the years I have become very organised and this helps. If you have disabilities, you really need to be organised. It reduces stress and pain if chores are done gradually and simplified.

Oct 15th

It was a beautiful day, just right for a bit of gardening before winter. Unfortunately, my role in gardening has diminished gradually over the last 50 years. I used to do it all; growing vegetables and flowers, the digging, pruning, weeding and mowing. Anything and everything. Now my role is just sharing in the design and choosing plants and minimal practical stuff. I do a little weeding and planting up pots and I love growing from seeds, but Keith does all the heavy stuff.

At the start of my RA, I was working in the park, and I was energetic and strong able to have a go at anything. How things change! I see so much in the garden that I would love to do if only I could, but I have to be patient and wait until Keith has a chance to do it. [especially hard as he works part time getting paid for doing other people's gardens!] It sometimes feels frustrating even after all this time when I just want to get on with stuff and I can't.

Oct 16th

Today I had a meeting for my volunteer role. It was a new venue, so I tried my best to research beforehand. There was only one blue badge space, all the council car parks work differently. Of course, when I arrived the space was gone so I parked and put my badge up and hoped for the best. Of course, having a blue badge does not always mean the parking is free, particularly in hospitals! Nowadays many machines are impossible for me to use due to my reduced hand function. Either I cannot get the ticket out or I cannot retrieve my payment card, or I get the registration number wrong! Sometimes you can use a phone which is easier for me but sometimes you need an app which I don't have. All this makes volunteering harder as I can only walk very small amounts now. Sometimes the parking is further away than the qualifying amount for obtaining a blue badge!

Sometimes everything is a fight.

Oct 17th

I was very excited today as I received a message saying that the photo that I took in Knaresborough last week had been chosen for the 'BBC Big picture'. I was amazed. This was wonderful for me and a great achievement as I love photography but like most things in my life there are restrictions in what I am able to take. My hand function does not allow me to be able to use manual settings or change lenses, so I need to keep it simple. My walking is limited to around 100 metres, and my standing is limited to about five minutes and of course I cannot get down onto the ground so I just try and be as creative as I can. I was using my scooter on this occasion, so this gave me a bit more choice of shot. Often, I have to drive, park where I can and shoot! This was the first time I have sent in a photo, so it really inspired me.

Later on, I looked on the healthunlocked website [for people with health difficulties] and noticed that there are issues with JAK Inhibitors such as Baricitinib which is the medication that I take to control my RA. Now apparently it's not issued to people over 65 or those with cardiac problems. Later on, I asked my rheumatologist about this and she said as I am monitored regularly with blood tests they would pick up problems and therefore it's safe for me to continue on it. There are always problems balancing medications though and I have to take about seven different ones. Most have side effects that may or may not affect you, Baricitinib can raise cholesterol, many drugs for pain are likely to cause constipation or cause addiction or both, tablets for hypertension can cause palpitations, swelling of ankles or dizziness. If I start a new drug, then I need to make sure that I notice any symptoms that occur.

Oct 18th

I have been preparing minestrone soup for a social group I attend. As is often the case I need to be organised and think ahead to ensure I can manage everything. Reaching ingredients can be a problem or cutting some vegetables or opening jars [although I have a good opener].

On this day I needed a container for the soup to be lifted down from a high cupboard. It had to be big enough but light so I could put it into a suitable bag that I was able to lift into the car. I did ok on this as I have a food processor, double handled pan that I can lift and right-angled chopping knife but I had to ensure my bottles of herbs had been opened though because they are too small for my various openers!

Today I received a telephone call to arrange the pre-assessment for the elbow replacement surgery. I have needed surgery on my right elbow since Aug 2021 when an x-ray revealed that all the cartilage had eroded, and the ulnar nerve was caught underneath and sometimes it gives me pain right from my elbow to my hand. I have been through six consultants! Fifteen months was spent attending two hospitals which actually do not even provide elbow replacement surgery! [3 consultants in those 2].

I have been attending the present hospital for almost a year now. I have seen two different consultants plus the neurologist/spinal specialist who had to check if the pressure on my spinal cord and stability of my neck would be safe for surgery. Another two months later and now I am at the pre-assessment stage! You can imagine the sheer frustration and anger I felt in the first two hospitals when I found out eventually after long waits that they couldn't do the surgery that I needed. In the present hospital they keep cancelling and rebooking appointments continually. Hopefully I will get the operation quite soon now.

Oct 19th

Grandkids were round here today. It is easier for me at my house where there are less games and toys to fall over and two tables where I can draw with them or do play doh or games. Also, I can get snacks and drinks myself. In other houses I feel disabled as my house is set up to suit me with adapted utensils and lots of seats and it's compact too. Today we played hide and seek, I was hiding, and I so wanted to be found. I really needed to sit down; I nearly had to shout out! When they were close, I jumped out at them [what a relief] and they shrieked!

Oct 20th

We met some friends for a meal in a carvery today. I don't usually go to carveries as you have to queue for food and serve yourself with vegetables, sauces and gravy. This is difficult for me with my very reduced hand function. I'm not keen on parties, pubs or anywhere that involves chatting in a group either. If you sit down or are sitting on a mobility scooter or in a wheelchair it can make you feel anti- social and you miss lots of the conversation and feel excluded. I try to circulate but then I need to sit down after five minutes so it just doesn't work. Now I'm older some gatherings have more seats so it's a bit easier to move around. Thats one advantage of ageing!

Oct 21st

Not much to record today. Just using my PC and doing some household chores. My role has diminished gradually over the years. I do shopping online, organise menus, do some of the meal preparation and cooking [there is a handy seat] and some washing up. I can only do a little cleaning and dusting, I cannot hoover now or change beds, and I gave up on ironing years ago! I don't miss doing any of these things though. I always hated changing beds and cleaning windows. I just have to make sure these things get done without me feeling that I am nagging. I have certainly learnt to be patient over the years.

Oct 22nd

Today I was clearing summer bedding plants from my pots and planting bulbs. I have to lift the compost in a small bucket and then I can manage. I use a seat but still get back pain after a few minutes of bending over so I limit myself to about 45 minutes at a session with lots of rests. I really love seeing the spring bulbs when they appear so it's all worth it.

Oct 23rd

We were looking after our six year old grandson today and we chose to go to a local museum with a Roald Dahl section. I researched ahead as usual as I needed to take my mobility scooter. It was amazingly accessible, and we could park on the yellow lines outside with my blue badge. The blue badge is such a help as parking gets harder and harder. I am actually an asset to friends and family when they come in my car! These days some places allow free carers and then there is the easier parking! It was a very enjoyable day but tiring looking after a six year old from 9: 30 to 6: 30.

Oct 24th

We went on a walk in our local area [me on my mobility scooter].

It was a Halloween trail, and it was pretty muddy in places. My disability scooter does not like muddy paths, and I have to take great care to avoid it as far as possible or I could easily get stuck. I can't go anywhere that might be muddy alone. Although obviously it's sometimes hard to predict but if I am caught out my mobility scooter has a good turning circle, so I have to turn around and go another way. Luckily it was National Trust parking today and disabled parking is free so no annoying machines to deal with.

On the way back home a light on the dashboard was telling me my boot was open and was intermittently beeping loudly. We had not opened the boot, so I don't know what was going on but sometimes the sensor has a mind of its own! Today it wasn't a problem as Keith got out and opened it and shut it firmly and that cures the problem but if I am by myself, I cannot do that as I cannot open the boot!

Once I was at the zoo, I had to flag down a passerby who helped me. At other times I have had to ignore it and drive to my destination and then get someone to do it for me. I got the garage to check it out but as it's intermittent no-one could find the fault, so I still have the problem.

Oct 25th

We thought our grandson would enjoy the cinema so we planned a visit but there were a few hitches for me. Firstly, there were very few disabled spaces and there are never any free at this cinema as they are often used by people without blue badges. There are no checks, so they get away with using them. I have mentioned this in the past, but nothing has ever changed. On this day I did manage to walk in from our parking space but in the foyer the only seats were for people using the cafes. I had to sit down, however, as my sciatica pain was severe after four minutes walking, so I had to sit in the cafe seats [although I wasn't eating or drinking]. Then we went in, I was in for another shock! I had assumed that the rows were numbered from the screen, and I had booked seats that I thought were quite near the front but that was not the case! In front of me was a gigantic staircase, fairly steep with about 40 steps [or so it seemed to me] so I made the choice to sit in some free seats at the front and hope for the best. I couldn't have climbed those steps to the top. Luckily, we didn't need to move, and our grandson loved the film.

Oct 26th

I had a chiropody appointment in the morning. Luckily for me there is a car park with a barrier for blue badge users only so I can drive independently for this appointment as I know that I can manage the very short walk in. I have to ask Keith to drive me to quite a lot of my appointments, particularly in hospitals, as you cannot be sure of close parking or indeed any parking.

In the afternoon we took our grandson to soft play and met with our middle daughter and our two tiny grandchildren. I would like to go into the play area with my small grandchildren but it is extremely difficult for me to walk without shoes so I can only watch and chat to them at the drink and snack break. Its quite annoying as I would love to be hands on.

Oct 27th

Today I really fancied peanut butter sandwiches for lunch and so

I was very annoyed to see the jar of peanut butter had run out and the new one was on the top shelf out of my reach! I did think of pushing it off the shelf with a long-handled spoon but thought I might not be able to catch it, and it would end up in hundreds of pieces on the hard kitchen floor! Usually, I can prepare my lunch and dinners independently but sometimes I need a little help. I have my own techniques for opening cans, packets and jars. I have to ensure that no-one loses my scissors or borrows them as they suit me when most others don't [My span is too limited to work most of them] I have an electric can opener, but I often just lever the ring pull and can lid off with a knife. I have a jar opener that is pretty good, but it doesn't work on plastic milk containers, so I have another opener for those! I keep things that I use regularly out on the worktop or in an easily accessible drawer.

Oct 28th

I was at home making cakes today. I don't do this often as I prefer not to use a food processor and so a short session is enough for my thumbs, wrists and elbows. I love to make chocolate chip cookies. They are so easy and quick and tasty. I use a processor for chopping nuts and I have two different whisks. I also have a light mixing bowl and pans. I just get stuck for lemon zests and have to get them prepared ahead unless Keith is in. It can be difficult to be spontaneous with RA.

Oct 29th

It was a tiring few days with one daughter and grandson staying and another daughter and grandchildren visiting. I was worn out and had to enlist lots of helpers for meal preparation and setting the table. I used to do all the food preparation but now I know my limits. I have always had to do some pacing and alternating of activities but now I can only stand a few minutes, so I have a handy chair and table in the kitchen.

Oct 30th

I played scrabble with my sister today. I struggle to get the box out of the cupboard but apart from that it's plain sailing unless I drop a letter! I have to get a dustpan and brush to pick up little things or flat pieces of paper off the floor. Obviously today I had help so it was no problem. I often use the dustpan and brush to brush pieces of puzzles or counters into their boxes or to collect rubbish when the kids have left stuff out on the table and rushed home.

Oct 31st

The last day of the diary and today my focus is on medication in child proof bottles. My neighbour came round today as she couldn't open her pill bottle. Luckily Keith was in, and he opened it for her, because I can't do them either! I haven't been able to open childproof tops since I was about 30 when I already had fused wrists and deterioration of finger joints and lots of stiffness. Sometimes the packs are difficult too as it takes strength in the fingers to push the pills out of the strips. Also, there are times when they suddenly shoot out like a catapult and end up on the floor! I usually have mine on a mini tray to reduce the chance of losing the tablets. There is no bottle opener as far as I'm aware that can open medication jars due to the double action i.e. push down while turning. I think they can be issued with normal tops though. I have not asked but according to google they can be!

This diary was written in October 2023 and in the spring of 2024, I reached my 50 year anniversary of living with RA. In the first chapter of this new book, I am returning to my early life before my RA started just to set the scene.

Chapter 1: Setting the Scene

I was born in the early fifties and my first ever home was a three-bed semi-detached house with a garden. There was a path nearby leading to a large common, complete with a river and willow trees as well as an interesting dump to explore!

Maybe it doesn't sound that idyllic, but it was a wonderful place for a child to live, although perhaps not very classy. There again, looking back it was unusual for working class people to own their own home at that time just after World War two. My parents only owned their own home because my mum sensibly used the money she received from the post office as a deposit. She was given the money when she was made to leave work due to getting married! A normal occurrence in 1947. We had a lovely big garden at the back and the front with bushes and grass. I used to play loads of ball games there, throwing a ball up the wall to bounce and catch, skipping and making camps.

I can remember being in the front garden and waiting to go outside and play with my friends. In those days we all knocked on neighbours' doors to play with the children nearby from a very young age. We lived on a corner and lots of children used to gather by the lamppost opposite our house and I remember we played marbles on the street, using the drain covers for the holes. We also played chase games, ball games and rode our scooters and bikes around the block. Near our house was the path leading to the common and that was my favourite place to go with friends. There was a playground on it and a huge area of grassy common, as well as the river and the dump! There were so many opportunities for play, we were never bored when the weather was fine.

By the river we climbed the willow trees, caught tiddlers in jars, paddled in the stream. In the playground we swung and climbed to our hearts content. The climbing frame was very high, I used to climb to the top and swing from the top bars by my legs. My mum must have been so scared although I don't remember her being there that much. The children just went off together in those days. I also jumped off the top by piling straw next to the climbing frame and then leaping off onto it. [There was no soft playgrounds then only hard concrete]. It is a wonder that children didn't have bad accidents, but I don't remember any. I can also remember the concrete tunnel that we used to jump on as well as sitting in to chat as we got older.

In fact, I was a bit of a climber and adventurer. I took after my mum and my nana! I know I used to climb on my auntie's garage roof when I was about 11 or 12. At home, I went off with my friend Claire and we explored the nearby fields and country lanes by bike or sometimes we went walking for miles. We used to cross over a thick pipe above the river to get to the fields on the other side. These were often boggy, I can remember getting my foot stuck in the mud and sinking down a few inches. Another time I lost a shoe in the river. We would go out after breakfast and only return for meals! I had a lovely childhood, and it was so much freer in those days.

At the weekends and holidays my dad used to drive us out into the countryside where we walked and climbed hills and had picnics or sometimes, we visited my nana and grandad. They had an incredibly long garden where they grew their own vegetables and fruit, my nana made lovely pies and cakes for tea.

Every year we had a holiday and stayed in a bed and breakfast in Norfolk so that I could enjoy the sandy beaches and play loads of ball games. Sadly, this all ended in 1961 when my dad died after a few weeks in hospital. He had had an operation for cancer but relapsed a few days later. I remember a local policeman coming to tell us as we had no phone at that time. I was nine years old; my mum was forty and she had to quickly find a job. I think I grew up quickly after this.

My adolescence did not last long either as I left school in July 1967 just before my 16th Birthday, and after my GCEs in June. At the end of the summer holidays, I started my first full time job in Barclays bank. I was happy to leave school as I wanted to earn my own money so I could buy a car, travel and get a flat in London. I also wanted money to go out more in the evenings and weekends with my friends. At the bank I worked on the accounting machines of that time and did junior office work. I was a general dogsbody really. I wanted to work as a cashier, but it would have taken me years. Only boys could move through the system quickly then. This is the first time that I began to get pain in my wrists and fingers, I will never know if that was the start of my RA.

Towards the end of my time at the bank I passed my driving test. Learning to drive was my first goal once I was earning a weekly wage. I wanted to get my own car and at the time this was quite unusual because only about 20% of women held driving licences then and they didn't all own cars. I was determined, I think because we had no car at home, not since I was 9 when my dad had died, so I saved every week and paid for about 12 lessons and by the age of 18 I had achieved my dream by buying a blue grey mini with a stripe down it. I loved it. After this I knew I wanted to change my job. Work was ok but not very fulfilling and when my friend Barbara got a new job at a publishing and printing company, she asked me if I wanted to apply for a job as a wages clerk there, so I did and I was accepted. This was a very cushy job. I typed up cash sheets on a proper typewriter, worked out the hours and overtime for the printers, worked out their tax and then made up paypacks with real money in envelopes! It was very laid back with no pressure but again not very challenging. It was so relaxed that I was told off for being too quick. They said they would run out of work! I can't imagine that happening these days! During this time, I was very healthy and there was no pain that I can remember.

After a couple of years working there, I decided to leave to go travelling to France and Spain with two friends, Claire and Rose. It wasn't possible to take a year out in those days and people didn't have gap years, holiday leave was only about three weeks a year, so I had to give in my notice in order to travel for two months. I also needed extra money for my trip and so I worked at Tesco's on the till on Saturdays. The Tesco money would have taken too long to save up and as I could earn a lot more by working in the Vauxhall car factory than I could by being a wages clerk, I got a job there on the production line. Quite weird really that Vauxhalls paid so much more. I saved up in a month and left. Off we went hitch-hiking through Europe for 6 weeks to France and Spain. I was full of energy and really excited to go.

When I returned from Europe, I need to find work quickly and luckily it was easily possible in 1970. First, I went to the labour exchange, as it was known then, and they booked me an interview at 11am for office work in the local laundry. At the interview the manageress asked me when I could start. I said that tomorrow or next week would be ok. She then said how about now! They gave me a coffee then I got started! I then found out why they were so desperate! The previous lady who was doing the accounts had become overwhelmed and there were unpaid bills and paperwork everywhere.

I also had to work at the switchboard, an old fashioned one with plugs, and sometimes I had to pretend to be the manager when the manager refused to come to the phone! Sometimes I took in the laundry when there was no-one else to do that. I only stayed there for about three months and then I did some temping. The trouble with temping is that the companies who needed temps were nearly always behind with their work and being in a new place and having to learn staff names and routines was tiresome. I wanted something more interesting and permanent.

While I was temping, I was applying for jobs in London as I wanted to achieve my ambition to share a flat and live there. In 1970 it wasn't that common for girls to move out of their home until they got married but I thought it would be exciting and there were too many restrictions for going out when I was living at home. Anyway, it didn't take long to get a job. I'm not sure if I applied for others but I completed an application to work as a computer operator.

At the end of 1970 there were only computers in a few large corporations or companies and the job I applied for was for the Post Office in Dollis Hill in north London and after six weeks I was offered the job. It was a great job. In those days the computers took up the whole room, which also had to be kept at an optimum temperature which was great as it was never too cold or hot. We just put up magnetic tapes for the users and sent messages via a terminal to check they were managing ok. The rest of the time we could chat and make toast and drinks.

I loved living in the city. It was exciting and busy with pubs and parties and clubs; it was very full on. Sometimes I felt so alive and so energetic that I went off for long walks. Once I remember suddenly driving off to Wales on my own just to explore. I stayed in youth hostels [although I had to pretend I wasn't driving, or they would not have let me in!].

I was living in London for about two years and then I got the travel bug again and planned an overland tour to Greece and the Greek Islands followed by a trip to Italy, Bavaria and Austria. I had a fantastic time travelling but then of course I had to return and find another job aged 20.

I found work in a nearby pub; I enjoyed this a lot as a stop gap to finding full time work. The memories I have are adding up loads of drink prices in my head, learning about cocktails and being invited out for drinks afterwards! After this I found a job as accounts clerk at a company that made time recorders [clocking in machines]. It was quite a boring job as there were periods when there was nothing to do and so I read my book which apparently, I was not allowed to do as I needed to pretend I was busy!

After all this time I was feeling that I really wanted a career as opposed to just working to make money. I wanted a new challenge, but I was not sure what to do. At that time most girls worked as secretaries, typists, teachers and nurses or in banks, offices, factories or shops. Most had babies before 25 and then didn't work at all.

The girls' grammar school that I had attended had helped me to focus on having a career and making me more aware of possibilities and my teachers had thought of options most of which involved training courses or university. Only a very small number of girls went to university then, in fact there were not many boys either. In 1970 about 14% of students went to university so you can bet that there was only about 5% of girls.

I liked teaching my sister Heather so I thought I might like to teach. In those days five O levels got you into a Teacher Training College if you passed the application, interview and written test. I decided to train at Nottingham and then I changed my plan when I met Keith, got married in the summer of 1973, and decided to do my training at Radlett in Hertfordshire instead. At this time, I was very fit and healthy and strong.

So, this was where I was in my life before everything changed. I was blissfully unaware of what was ahead and had many plans for the future. I enjoyed being out and about with my friends and having fun, trying new activities, walking, playing sports, travelling in the UK and beyond and I definitely wanted a career too. After all I was only 22.

Chapter 2: The First Decade; The Start of my RA!

It was the spring of 1974. I was in the gym doing P.E. with the kids in my class as part of a teaching practise. At the end of the session, I was shaking my hands out with the children for the end of the exercises and that's when it suddenly hit me. I just couldn't shake them out! My wrists would not move; I just could not shake them at all. At that time, I played piano and that felt all wrong too. I was due to play in assembly soon, but I was way too scared to do that, so I just threw a sickie.

Anyway, I got through the summer term and in the holidays, I had managed to get a temporary job in the local park. I was very keen to do this as it was outside work on the playing fields and looking after the gardens and this suited me down to the ground. I had always loved sport, and I was often outside walking the countryside with dogs whenever I got the chance.

In this job I had to drive the tractor to cut the grass, seed the football pitches, trim the edges of the bowling greens and look after the rose gardens. Also being a young woman of 22 I was always being told to make tea [that was women's work in those days!] The tea was in a massive pot; I could barely lift it. It was the hardest thing I had to do when I was working there. I could manage all the rest of the work, although I did have terrible stiffness in my hands and feet in the mornings, and I had to walk through the pain. I can recall some of the men making fun of me when I made tea. I was reinforcing their stereotypes that women were not very strong and generally a bit pathetic. In fact, I had always been physically strong and would have easily managed all of this work a few months before. It upset me a lot and dealing with the pain as well was very challenging, although I did still love that job, and continued through the holidays as mostly I worked independently or with one person. I just hoped the pain would disappear soon.

At night I struggled to sleep, I can remember putting my hands under the pillows to try and ease the pain. At that time, I could not really understand why I had such difficulty lifting things or why my wrists would not flex properly. I wasn't sure what to do about it. I just hoped it would go away, and I could go back to being the person I was before.

I returned to college to get on with my course and consulted my doctor about the pain and stiffness. He gave me Ibuprofen, this helped to reduce my symptoms to a degree, but he did not give me the answers I needed so I still did not know what was happening to me. That term I became disenchanted with the teaching and was not really sure if it was the right choice for me. By sheer coincidence I had a hernia operation in the Christmas break and after the anaesthetic, along with a stay in hospital, which was three or four days in the seventies, I came home and recovered from the operation. During this time, I decided to give the course up. I have often wondered was it the removal of the stress of the course that sent me into remission or the complete physical rest after the operation or the anaesthetic or a combination? Anyway, whatever it was, the pain mysteriously disappeared! I just forgot about pain, found myself a new job in a children's home and got on with my life.

During the next four years I was fit and healthy. I worked at the children's home for more than two years as a housemother and I was doing a whole lot of physical work. I was looking after the children and cooking for eight, doing household chores, bathing children, playing with them and supervising them. I still wasn't sure what I wanted to do for a career though, so I decided to go back to college to take two A levels and work part time. I had left school after passing 6 GCE's [as they were then!] but I had no higher qualifications. I had been working since my 16th birthday and now I needed a new direction as it wasn't going to be teaching. I just didn't know what it would be!

At the end of 1977 when I was 26, my career plans went on hold when our first daughter was born. She was so beautiful and amazing; we were so happy. Everything was going so well and then five months later the pain in my fingers, wrists and elbows returned and it became difficult to put on tiny clothes and lift carrycots and prams. I didn't want to take medication as I was breast feeding and this was working very well and so I coped with the pain as well as I could. Being a mother became harder, but I carried on feeding for another four months until I decided that I needed something to take away all this stiffness and pain.

Once again, I was restarted on Ibuprofen and again it did take away my pain but I still had no idea that during these times of pain, inflammation and stiffness I was irreparably damaging my joints. Any non-steroidal anti-inflammatory drugs [NSAIDs] reduce the symptoms but do not stop the disease. The joints settled down after a few more months though and I was able to reduce and then stop the tablets and I felt like myself again. I was in remission for the second time.

I so enjoyed the time with my baby daughter, we wanted to have another child and so in 1980 we had our second wonderful, smiley, baby daughter. I now had a demanding two year old and a very hungry baby who wanted food every two hours and it was very tiring for me but also wonderful having the privilege to be with them both as they grew and developed. I had never thought that the pain and stiffness would return, but it soon did with a vengeance, and so when my baby was about five or six months old, I was forced to stop breast feeding and had to take anti-inflammatory tablets again and my pain and stiffness reduced. This time I did became more concerned and I worried about what was wrong, but I was still unaware of my diagnosis, so I got on with my busy life looking after my little ones and studying for an Open University degree in the evenings.

I did not work at that time, so I had the lion's, no, the lioness's, share of the parenting! [Incidentally, why do we have an expression 'the lion's share' when the lionesses actually do most of the work not the lions!]. I looked after my two little girls, did the household chores, cooking and shopping as well as taking our dog out every day and I did quite a lot of the gardening too. That's the way it was for many families in the seventies and eighties; men were employed full time and women with babies and young kids most often became full time mothers and housewives.

We really wanted a third baby, but I was struggling with tiredness a lot of the time. I can remember going out to sleep in our VW camper one night because I was so tired. My husband Keith was sleeping in the house so that I would not be disturbed. I remember this happening because I just could not get to sleep at all that night! There were owls hooting and cats walking on the roof and I was just too strung up and desperate to sleep, however, amazingly that night no-one woke up in the house and so Keith got to sleep, I was even more tired! Anyway, I managed to convince myself that the reduced sleep and tiredness would only be for a short period and so we went ahead and in 1982 our third child was born. A sweet and placid baby girl.

Now I really had my hands full. Two small pre-school children and one baby and a dog. I was so busy that I even employed a cleaner for a few weeks but then she left for a better paid job, I did not replace her, so my house was never tidy. It was always full of toys and crafts and books all over the place during the daytime. I was incredibly well and happy during all the pregnancies, although during the third one I had a mouth full of ulcers due to extreme tiredness. There was no sign of RA at all though and I thought and really hoped that all the pain and stiffness had gone but of course it hadn't. It recurred in exactly the same way as before when my new baby daughter was around five or six months old.

The pain and stiffness and inflammation returned, mostly in my hands, and it was hard to dress the little ones and very painful to play with them in the hands-on way that I wanted to[excuse the pun!]. Most of the pain was in my fingers and wrists and elbows at this time. Lifting my toddlers and babies around was very difficult and there's so much lifting with little toddlers and babies. It's both a physically and mentally demanding role being a full-time mum.

Of course, now I know that this is generally what happens when women with RA have babies but back then I was oblivious to all this as I was not even aware that I had RA. Even if I had known I probably wouldn't have been warned about the likely recurrence after pregnancies at that time, as this was only realised later on. Also, there was not the range of drugs available to take safely while you were conceiving or pregnant at that time except possibly Sulphasalazine. [A disease modifying drug DMARD]. Nowadays there is lots of information on which drugs you can continue, and which ones should be stopped before pregnancy is even considered.

The thing that most concerned me back then was worrying about what the problem was with my hands and elbows and also feeling awful if one of my daughters grabbed me or knocked me at the wrist or elbow. I did not want them to be upset that they had hurt me. I had to try really hard not to scream out though because anyone holding me around my wrists or knocking my elbow or hands really hurt me and my immediate reaction was to cry out. By the time I was 30 some of the cartilage in my joints was already being eroded and I had lost most of the movement in my wrists and some in my elbows, finger joints and toes as well.

In some ways it was good not to know my diagnosis back then as I never had to make the decision about whether to have children or how many to have. On the other hand, I probably would have chosen to have three children anyway and I would have been started on Sulphasalazine and then I would probably have had a lot less damage in my joints now than I actually have. Indeed, consultants I see now often like to tell me, that it is only people like me who have had RA for many, many years that have hand deformities and need elbow replacements! I was born too soon! I am really glad though that RA treatments and surgery have improved so much over the last 50 years and that younger people with RA will be able to continue to live the life they want with maybe only a few adjustments. They probably will not need to make as many of the changes and adaptations that I have continually had to make in my life. Also, without a diagnosis or treatment I was doing all the wrong things as I had no advice, information or guidance and there was no internet then!

I was always carrying heavy babies and toddlers and lifting pushchairs, prams and highchairs. I also walked them all out most days with our dog, rain or shine unless it was pouring. A baby and two toddlers to dress with the dog waiting patiently for his walk. Coats, jumpers and shoes to put on. It exhausts me to even think about it now! When we returned the dog was often dirty and the kids needed undressing, and everyone was hungry!

Daily I had to struggle with nappies, clothes and tiny shoes and one of the hardest things to do was laces in shoes [no Velcro then] and putting the girls' hair into bunches and ponytails. I was cooking all the meals and snacks with a lot heavier pans than I have now and doing all the washing in a twin tub! I so loved all the things we did together though, the daily walks with our dog and playground visits, the crafts and drawing and painting and all the pretend play! It is physically demanding though and hard work on your joints and I didn't know anything about energy conservation, pacing and joint protection back then. We did read lots of books together though which allowed some rest, and we had a bit of TV time [although there were very few programmes for children back then in the Eighties]. I also I gave up the pram when my middle daughter was one and stuck to a pushchair and sling which was easier, and we were lucky to have our own car, me and the girls. If I had known what I know now I would have taken much more care but luckily for me although I had RA, I was very healthy and strong which I guess is a bit of a contradiction in some ways but then a strong immune system fights off infections even if it destroys joints as well!

Chapter 3: The Second Decade; The Diagnosis

Anyway once my children were 1, 3 and 5 I decided that enough was enough. I knew I would need to go to the doctor and ensure that I got answers to my questions this time and not just accept anti-inflammatory medication with no explanation of what was causing my symptoms. I wanted to know why my wrist could not move much, why my arms would not straighten and why I had such pain and stiffness every day.

I visited my G.P. Again, I was given NSAIDs but this time I asked all the questions that I had inside my head, I succeeded in getting a referral to see a rheumatologist. In my first appointment with the rheumatology consultant, I explained all my symptoms and was given a blood test. On the next appointment with the consultant, I was given the diagnosis...sero-positive rheumatoid arthritis [RA]. Sero-positive means you are positive for the rheumatoid factor [however you can still have RA without being positive and you can be positive and not have RA!] To give a diagnosis the consultant considers signs and symptoms and inflammatory markers in the blood as well as the test for the rheumatoid factor.

I remember this appointment very well as my consultant was very blunt and told me in no uncertain terms that my fingers and wrists would fuse so to make sure I used my hands in the correct positions because then I would still be able to use my hands when this happened! There was no hope in the way that he told me, and he didn't suggest any DMARDs at that time [Disease modifying anti-rheumatoid drugs that slow down the RA]. This of course meant that the rheumatoid continued to be active in my body even though my symptoms were better controlled.

I was devastated by this diagnosis. It was such a shock. I had been thinking there would be a way of making me better. I was so young, and I had always been healthy and fit and active. I never really got ill. I went away and talked about my situation to Keith and to all my friends and family, probably bored them to death, but I needed a way to get to grips with this, to get used to having a chronic condition that had no cure. When you have this sort of diagnosis you feel worried about the future you will have, you wonder whether you will be able to do the things that you are planning and if you will be able to manage to care for your children.

How different this would be these days. If it was now, I would have had x-rays, blood tests, maybe an MRI scan. Possibly I would have been put on a short-term steroid to knock out the inflammation quickly and then I would have been started on a disease- modifying antirheumatic drug to reduce the ongoing disease and of course the pain and stiffness. I would also have be given a leaflet with information and maybe a referral to an Occupational Therapist [OT] or a Clinical specialist nurse. Then there is also NRAS, a brilliant organisation for people with RA which wasn't around in 1983. NRAS stands for the National Rheumatoid Arthritis Society.

'NRAS was founded in 2001 by Ailsa Bosworth MBE, who now acts as the NRAS National Patient Champion having led the charity as CEO for 18 years.'[2] Ailsa started running this organisation from a room in her house and it has developed its services and information and guidance over the years. It is the only patient led organisation in the UK specialising in RA and Juvenile Idiopathic Arthritis [JIA] for under 16s. It supports, educates and campaigns for people with RA and their families. It has a daily helpline, many informative booklets, a self-management programme online and an online forum for members as well as stories and news on social media like Facebook, Instagram and a YouTube channel.

Back in 1983 I did my best to find out what I could about RA by reading books and asking questions but there wasn't much information around then, I had never heard of it, nor had my friends and so I was in the dark a bit. Even today people think RA is an old person's disease or they think it's a bit of arthritis or rheumatism when actually it is a chronic inflammatory autoimmune disorder. People of any age can be diagnosed with RA and the most likely time is 30-50 but there is also the juvenile form too for young people under 16.

The immune system is an intricate mechanism that enables our body to defend itself against bacteria, viruses and other organisms that want to invade it. A healthy immune system knows which particles are foreign to the body and which ones belong. In order to protect the body, it will attack outsiders that

---

[2] Foxton, P (2025) nras.org.uk

do not belong. The body also protects itself when there is damage caused by an accident resulting in a burn or a broken bone. In this case inflammation occurs as a necessary part of the repair process. In RA something goes wrong, and the immune system attacks its own joints.

This can happen gradually and slowly or often there are flare ups of one or many joints. During a flare up of RA the synovial lining of the joint becomes inflamed although it is not known what triggers the inflammation. The synovial fluid that lubricates the joint, keeping the cartilage slippery, is overproduced. The lining of the joint becomes thicker, and the cartilage begins to be destroyed. The cartilage normally acts as a shock absorber between the bones, so there will be more pain on movement when it starts to be destroyed.

Eventually if it is all destroyed the bones will fuse together, preventing the joint from working at all. Even if the bones do not fuse together the increased amount of fluid in and around the joint means that the joints become swollen and feel uncomfortable, this restricts movement at the joints even before actual damage occurs.

The joint capsule and ligaments also become stretched and loose, this leads to unstable joints and possibly deformities. As well as the joints internal body systems can also be affected and inflamed, and it can feel like having flu. Sometimes though, there is a remission, and the flare ups calm down for a while.

I had to come to terms with the fact that I now had an autoimmune condition that would likely affect all my joints but could also potentially affect my energy, my heart and lungs and other body systems as well as my body image and attractiveness to my husband. I sometimes worried that I wasn't what he bargained for when we met in 1972 and married in 1973. Luckily my RA was in remission on and off for quite a few years in my twenties and thirties and when it relapsed the pain and stiffness was controlled with NSAIDs. I was also fortunate that I didn't suffer from fatigue, apart from what was normal for a mum with three tiny children under five.

Fatigue does affect a large proportion of people with RA though. In a survey conducted by NRAS in 2014 '40 % of those surveyed said that they experienced severe and persistent fatigue.'[3] Fatigue is exhaustion, when you feel completely drained of energy, and sometimes it can feel like wading through treacle. It can be hard to do even the basics of life. It is more like having flu and is a lot worse than tiredness.

I have felt like that when I have had flare ups but fortunately not on a regular basis. It can last for days, weeks or months. NRAS advises that there is no one reason why many people experience fatigue but there is a lot of factors that may well cause it. These are pain, tiredness due to poor sleep, low mood and disease activity. Pain feels as if it drains your energy. It's harder to get on with things when you have pain and often everything takes longer and takes more out of you. It can sometimes lower your mood too so it's important to find ways to reduce pain that work for you.

My way of coping with pain I think must have been distraction, kids and babies tend to absorb all your time, energy

---

[3] Rheumatoid Arthritis and Fatigue (2014) nras.org.uk/resource

and thoughts. I did have periods of remission in between the periods of pain and stiffness, I did not spend much time thinking about me and my problems but only how to manage everything! Every day I got on with my busy life with my family and kept my career goals alive by doing an Open University degree in the evenings and the occasional 30 minutes I could find in the day. My eldest daughter says she just remembers doing lots of crafts, painting, pretending games, going on walks and visiting playgrounds. Also, she says she heard me sometimes scream out but didn't take much notice. It was obviously me pushing or knocking a joint that didn't work. Apparently, she wasn't worried by it!

Of course, there was the occasional time when my mind settled on negative future scenarios like what if I ended up in a wheelchair, or what if I wouldn't be able to do lots of the things that I wanted to do. I was always making plans for my life and they didn't involve having a disability! The trouble is that when you attend rheumatology appointments many of the people there will be those with the most severe problems. The people in remission or with less symptoms would be there less often, and this can lead to catastrophising. Also, when you attend hospitals, it always starts you off thinking about how the RA has messed things up for you and about all the things you might miss out on.

Not long after I was diagnosed, I had just started learning the clarinet because it was getting difficult to play my piano due to my loss of wrist movement. I can remember playing songs for my little ones to sing but I was reduced to very basic melodies which was fine for them, but it was clear I couldn't go back to playing classics. I loved the clarinet, so I changed instruments but after a couple of years I had to buy an adapted version with hole covers so that I didn't make excruciating squeaks when I played in a local band!

Meanwhile I loved to play badminton, and I wanted to play at a higher level but having no wrist action is not great for badminton! I did continue to play until my mid-forties though as it was such fun.

Of course, going to appointments at this time was certainly not fun! Early on I had two or three of my little ones with me and I always had to go loaded with paper, pencils, stickers and books to keep them amused. It wasn't unusual to wait for an hour to see the consultant. By the time I got in to see him it became difficult to remember what I wanted to ask! I had to start writing out lists beforehand to ensure that I remembered what was important. I still do that to this day because it's all too easy to be dismissed before you've thought of everything. It's also important to remember it is a consultation and decisions should be made after discussing the pros and cons. You have a say in what happens and it's essential to remember this. Make sure that things are explained properly and if you're not clear then ask.

Generally, consultants can give good guidance and listen to what you have to say but unfortunately consultants vary. They most likely have a lot of knowledge, hopefully some experience but they do not always have the ability to listen in a way that makes you feel heard and they are often in a rush. This means that you need to make sure that you get answers to the things that worry you and guidance and explanations about available options that may help so that you can decide how to go forward.

I always remember when I went for a consultation about hand surgery and the consultant looked in a horrified way at my hands and said something along the lines of 'those are wrecked, we can't do anything about those!' He really upset me, and I actually made a complaint about it as he was so rude and disrespectful. When questioned by the complaints department he said he was joking to which I replied that for some people this could have been deeply upsetting and although I knew I had some deformity and damage I did not like his attitude, it was disrespectful. I felt he should have had more empathy and understanding. If you are not satisfied though you can always get your GP to refer you for a second opinion.

It is also important to understand as much as you can about your condition and what you can do yourself to help manage your condition. No-one knows what causes RA and it's likely to be more than one factor. It seems that certain disposing factors in your genes make you more susceptible, but it's not directly inherited, other environmental triggers are needed too. Something like a virus or infection or it could be triggered by a trauma or stress and smoking is a risk factor as well. Probably it's a combination of two or three of these.

Whatever it is it cannot be changed [at present anyway] and so it's best to learn how to live in harmony with the diagnosis by respecting it and making concessions with how you live your life. Do not give up on living a rewarding and happy life though even if that life is a bit different from what you expected. Also, remember that nowadays, the management of RA is very good, far better than it was 40 years ago or even 20 years ago, and although there is no cure, most people diagnosed today can expect to lead pretty full and active lives once their disease is under control.

At this time during my late twenties and thirties I was learning with the Open University [OU] which was a fantastic organisation and probably still is. I could spread my learning over time, and it took me about nine years to complete my six modules to obtain my degree! I couldn't do any modules when the babies were in their first years, but I could do more when they went to nurseries and school. I remember the first time I went to an OU summer school at Reading University when I was 28 and I was dismayed to find that all the teapots and coffee pots were so heavy that I just could not pour them out. I didn't know anyone, and my disease was fairly invisible then and I just couldn't bring myself to ask for help so I had to drink whatever I could pour out. I couldn't be asking when I was 28 looking about 22!

Of course, over my life I have got used to asking for help, but it is a problem when you first encounter things and there wasn't such a thing as accessibility then. Nowadays there would be a form to complete, and assistance provided at a venue like this, however, people aren't always totally comfortable with saying they have a problem even if help is available.

Thinking back to this time, in my thirties, I think I was lucky to have our children fairly young, although, in fact, 26 for a first baby was actually later than average at that time in the late seventies. I rarely caught anything, and I was strong and I can remember swinging the girls round by my hands, giving them piggybacks, playing chasing games and walking in the countryside. Playing tug of war with the dog and doing lots of cooking together. Also scrabbling around on the floor where little kids spend most of their time. Also we had a twin tub washing machine which meant a lot of heavy wet washing to lift. I can still recall when we bought our first automatic one and the girls were fascinated watching their cuddlies spinning round and I was in my early thirties then. I was really happy back then, at home with the girls, but I still wanted a career when they were all at school and I wasn't sure what do.

At 35 I had nearly completed my OU degree, but I had completed modules in a wide range of subjects; science, genetics, social science, psychology, world religions, food technology and the Earths' resources and so I still wasn't sure what I could do with those! I had still been having flares every couple of years since the birth of my last daughter when I was 30.

I went to see my consultant and he finally suggested Disease Modifying Anti Rheumatic Drugs [DMARDs]. Back then there was only Gold and Sulphasalazine and maybe Methotrexate and I was started on Sulphasalazine. It made a massive difference to me. My symptoms disappeared and the registrar referred me to an Occupational Therapist [OT]. He was aware of OTs as his wife was the OT, but I didn't know then that this referral would change my life in so many ways.

My OT Marian was the first medical professional who took the time to explain things to me and really listen to me. Both of these things are extremely important, and they made a world of difference to me at that time. Marian assessed me fully by taking my history and present symptoms as well as listening to how I was feeling and how I was coping with things in my life. She asked about my medications and measured the range of movements in my joints and then asked me if I had any problems. She also checked how much pain I was experiencing. She was thorough and holistic and always gave me as much time as I needed. After this, during the sessions we spent together, she told me about the different types of medications that were around then [late 80s/early 90s]. There are analgesics, non-steroidal anti-inflammatory drugs known as NSAIDs, steroids, and of course disease modifying drugs known as DMARDS. She told me how to take them and also, she explained about side effects.

Everyone with RA will have some degree of pain and inflammation and stiffness some of the time so the first group of medications used for RA are analgesics like Paracetamol, Co-codamol and other pain medications. These should be used when the pain is worse.

Secondly, we discussed the NSAIDs, which are good at reducing inflammation and relieving pain. The pain relief can often be felt straight away but full pain relieving takes up to a week and occasionally longer. They need to be taken consistently for longer to reduce inflammation. Only one type should be taken at a time. NSAIDs must be taken with or just after food to protect your stomach. They should also be gastro-resistant and slow release is generally better. Preferably they should not be taken for long periods as they may cause problems to your stomach or oesophagus [as they did many years later for me].

Thirdly, she explained about steroids, used to reduce inflammation quickly at the start of treatment and to treat flares. Once the DMARD medication is in place the steroids should not be needed except for flares. They should always be taken for the shortest time at the lowest necessary dose due to their side effects [like osteoporosis]. If you have taken them for more than a month and you want to stop them then you need to lower the dose gradually as instructed by your doctor or consultant. They are sometimes given as a one-off injection.

Of course, the most important type of medication for RA then and now are the DMARDs. There are many different types these days and they all aim to control the disease, dampen it down and thus prevent damage to joints and organs by keeping inflammation under control. The development of new types of DMARDS will be discussed in the final chapter but when I started to take them in the late 1980s/early 1990s there was only Sulphasalazine and Methotrexate. Of course, medication is the best way to control your RA but there are other strategies that help with controlling pain, stiffness and flares and these will be discussed later.

Marian told me about the correct postures that would help to reduce my pain and also told me all about joint protection and how to use my joints in the best way to preserve my hand function as long as possible and reduce the chance of deformities. There is information about joint protection and posture in the Appendix. She also showed me hand exercises that I could do daily to help me to maintain the strength and functioning in my hands as well as general exercise to keep my muscles strong and maintain stamina.

She talked about the best shoes and clothing to wear and about equipment that might be useful for me in the kitchen. We also talked about social situations, asking for help and relationship issues and many other things that came up in our discussions including pain management. There are many things that you can do to help yourself to manage your pain and gain more control over your condition. NRAS now have online modules about many different areas of self-management for RA. This program is called SMILE-RA, and the modules are free to access on their website.

Of course, this was not available for me then but luckily, I had an excellent OT instead. I gradually gained information and knowledge over the years until eventually I became an expert patient and indeed all of us can become experts of our own particular RA because we all have a different experience of RA and our pain is also unique to each of us. Anyone with RA is unlikely to be pain free but we have to learn how to turn the volume down by whatever means we can and everything that I learnt has helped me to do this. Anyway, I was so impressed by my OT that I decided that this was the career that I wanted. I could really help other people with RA and other medical conditions in the same way that Marian helped me.

At this time in my life my children were getting older, but I still needed to be very active and strong and physically able as well as being very organised. At 36 my children were 4, 6 and 8, two at school and one at nursery. We loved being active and going for days out picnics with hide and seek, bike rides to the pub, climbing trees and making dens in the woods, swimming, ball games, playgrounds and loads of dog walking. It was during this time that my middle finger joints started to deteriorate, and my fingers started to drift into ulnar deviation. This is where your fingers bend towards your little fingers on each hand. RA is symmetrical so what happens to one hand or wrist, or elbow will almost certainly happen to the other [in small joints anyway]. Once this damage to my fingers happened it made it more difficult to do sewing or knitting, crafts, playing instruments or opening jars or locks on doors.

I can remember being in a restaurant and going into the toilet, locking the door and then becoming trapped when I just could not open the door! I gradually panicked more and more and began to shout. It was a small place, and the toilet was near the staff kitchen and eventually someone heard and between us we managed to get the door open.

Since that time I always have to assess toilets before I lock them. This means that I often can't risk locking them at all and I have to stick a bag or my foot near the door. Sometimes though, people can still push the door open and then they are embarrassed and surprised to see me and I am embarrassed and very apologetic as well, but what choice do I have? This could all be a lot better if all toilets had the locking systems that some disabled toilets have, the 'lift to lock' disabled toilet mortice door locks or disabled toilet indicator bolt sets or similar. These all have easy turn handles and are not so tight and fiddly to use. If all toilets had these it would make my life so much easier. More recently I have been using disabled toilets but even these are variable too.

Another thing that was difficult then and now was opening jars [with no wrist movement] I remember making mince pies one Christmas and having made the pastry I just could not open the jar of mincemeat. No-one else was in so I stuck the jar into the door hinges but that didn't work [and even when it does it takes the paint off]! so eventually I had to take the jar to the next-door neighbour to get the top off. It was so frustrating and annoying. Actually, nowadays, I have a pretty good jar opener which opens all sizes of jars and bottles except plastic milk containers.

It was also harder to clean things in the kitchen but somehow, I managed by doing activities that were hard on my hands like cleaning, baking and gardening for short periods. I could never blitz tasks. The medication was working quite well at this time but after a couple of years I gradually reduced them but of course my body did not like this and went into a flare so eventually after a few months I had to restart the Sulphasalazine again and I stayed on it for a long time after this. Once I was ok again, I finished my OU degree and a year later at 37 I found myself a job in an activity centre for people with severe learning disabilities and challenging behaviour, not the easiest of jobs for me, but the closest I could find to being an OT!

I also went to visit two OT departments and spent an hour or two learning about what the OTs did and luckily for me an OT assistant job came up in one of them two months after I had started the Learning Disabilities job. I applied and was accepted. This is when my career in OT started.

Chapter 4: The Third Decade; Working Life

I was working part time as an assistant supporting OTs in various departments with people who had had strokes and heart attacks. I also worked in the hand injuries and general medical wards with people who had amputations, suffered trauma, or anyone who needed rehabilitation really. I loved it. It was so different from anywhere I had worked before or anything I had done.

I was a bit worried though, about whether I would be able to manage to support people with strokes or push people in wheelchairs or help people to stand and position themselves, due to my reduced hand function. We also lifted people, to transfer them back then, but actually I managed all of this safely and with no problems. Also, with it being an OT department there was more understanding of my abilities and my limits so it all went well and after a while I decided to start a full time OT course. The nearest training centres were London or Northampton. I chose the latter.

At the time my children were 13, 11 and 9 so fairly independent but I employed someone to do some ironing and housework and just to be there with them after school in case they needed any help. This helped me as well as I wanted to be able to manage the course physically and mentally. I drove daily four days a week sharing the driving with another mature student [I was 40 then]. I really loved learning, OT has such diverse areas of study both theory and practical. There were three placements where you worked full time in an OT department and lots of learning, exams, assessments and essays. It was hard work, so much to cover; nerves and muscles to learn, anatomy, human biology, psychiatry, psychology, management, counselling, theory of OT and activity analysis. My body held up surprisingly well and I only struggled with the excess of writing, the note taking, essays and exams and also with carrying books [This was the early nineties, so we did not use internet or kindles then!]. Later on, I was given extra time in exams and an amanuensis[scribe] to write for me, a very strange experience in an exam, but it did help me.

The scariest thing was learning about RA. I had never really realised at this point that our body systems could be affected as well as our joints when you have RA and I hadn't really thought through any worst scenarios, as they were at that time, probably because I wanted to think about best case scenarios!

At lectures we were shown, what seemed to me, photos of horrific results; of complications or joint deformities and at one point I remember walking out. It just upset me so much. I just couldn't deal with it. The main complications nowadays are inflammation of the lungs or the tissues around the heart, inflammation of the eyes or blood vessels, carpal tunnel syndrome, problems in the cervical area of the spine and osteoporosis but many of these are unlikely to happen and if they do it will be later in life.

Normally the most likely problems are joint damage to the bone and cartilage, damage to the tendons and maybe some deformities, although these are much less likely now that treatments and surgery are so much better at controlling the inflammation and replacing joints. The only thing I had experienced at this time was dry eyes apart from the joint damage to my wrists, elbows and fingers but at that time, the early 1990s, there was no surgery available to correct or repair these joints or if there was, I wasn't offered it. Of course there is now. Ironically, it's not needed as much nowadays with better and more effective medications and much more available information. The medication I did receive, and my knowledge about managing my condition, allowed me to complete my course and obtain my OT Degree. Then I had to find a job.

I was lucky, I was able to train in a job that I loved that actually was a good fit with my RA as the variety of activities meant that I didn't put a strain on any particular joint and there were active parts and sedentary assessments and admin, so a mixture of both physical and cognitive tasks. I was also lucky as there were grants and no fees then in the early 1990s and by saving when I had been working, I was able to train full time and pay for the support after school.

Lots of people with RA.won't be able to do this now and may well need to work in situations that are less suitable and so it's important to know all about the Disability Discrimination Act.

Under Disability law, derived from the Equalities Act 2010, it is unlawful for employers to discriminate against employees [or jobseekers] with disabilities. If you are in work and have problems that make it difficult for you to remain in work, and you have a disability like RA then these problems may be solved with reasonable adjustments. Your employer has a legal duty to make reasonable adjustments to enable you to continue to work.

These reasonable adjustments might be some of the following: allowing flexible working hours or shorter hours, the provision of aids such as screen reading software or it could be adaptations to premises or at your workstation, adapting workplace policies, reviewing job duties and making changes or allowing time off for medical appointments. You could probably suggest your own ideas that could help you as long as they are acceptable to other staff and the management. You could request an OT assessment to help you with ideas and if necessary, an 'Access to Work' assessment. An OT will take a holistic approach to help you suggest reasonable adjustments and support you with your employers.

Access to Work can help with providing a grant for specialist equipment and assistive software, support workers, like a travel buddy or an assistant at work, the costs of travelling to work if you cannot use public transport, adaptations to your vehicle so you can get to work or physical changes to your workplace.

I had Access to Work to provide a suitable chair with adjustable height and arms. It was set up for me to use at the correct height for my desk. Correct sitting posture is very important when you have RA and it helps reduce pain. The computer screen should be straight ahead when you are sitting straight up with you back supported. You should not need to look down. The seat should be at the correct height so that your elbows are in line with the top of the desk and armrests may help too. The only trouble was that I worked part time and then the chair tended to go walkies! I could not alter it myself so once I had tracked it down, I had to ask some kind person to reset it. Eventually I wrote a sign saying, 'hands off', however it still sometimes disappeared. I also had an electric hole punch that everyone was envious of and my own electric fire as I had, and still have, a terrible circulation and a touch of Renaulds disease.

The other assessment I also had at that time was for a new door entry system as a new one was going to be installed at the entrance to our building. The planned one would have proved very difficult for me as it was not possible for me to turn a knob and press at the same time. I would have been unable to get in at all. There were no press button disability access doors then. I can't actually remember what the solution was back then, but I was consulted so that we could find a system that would work for me and everyone else.

If you think creatively, think about anything that makes your life more of a challenge than it would be for a person without a disability then hopefully you'll get a good result. Obviously, this does depend on the situation and how helpful your manager is, however, at least there is a legal right to reasonable adjustments now. I also remember having my own wheeled container with my files to save me lifting heavy things. Maybe you would not need those now either as we live in a digital world but as far as I can see the NHS and GPs still seem to use letters, text, telephone and email correspondence as well as digital recording on databases so maybe it would be needed if you cannot open drawers or lift heavy things.

It might be preferable to reduce your hours or change jobs if your work is too demanding though or if some areas of your job are causing pain or fatigue or if you physically cannot manage even with adjustments. If you find yourself in financial difficulties after reducing hours, then you may be able to receive universal credit to top up your income. You will need to work at least 30 hours if you are under 60 or over 16 hours if you have a disability or are over 60. Under the Equality Act of 2010 [4] 'If you have a physical or mental impairment that has a 'substantial' and 'long-term' negative effect on your ability to do normal daily activities then you have a disability.' There is of course a financial assessment taking into account your present income and outgoings and also those of your partner if you have one.

If you want to apply for a new job, it's probably worth noting whether the company and job you are applying for has the disability confident symbol on the application. If it has then you are guaranteed an interview for jobs that are advertised with this symbol provided you meet the basic requirements of the job. Nowadays you will not normally be asked about your health and medical issues unless you are offered the job. The only exceptions being where there is an essential part of the job that the employer has to know the applicant will be able to manage. They also may ask if there needs to be any adjustments for the interview.

Having said that if you are starting a new job, it is usually better to be up front about your medical situation. If you do not disclose your condition and you need reasonable adjustments

---

[4] Definition of Disability under the Equality Act (2010) gov.uk/definition-of-disability-under-equality-act-2010

later on, then the employer does not need to provide them if they have been unaware of your condition and how it effects your working day.

Anyway luckily when I started work as an OT, I could pretty much manage most things. The only help I had to request was lifting heavier items and there was usually some wonderful admin person around to help. I do remember that when I was assessing people, they often noticed the deviation of my fingers and they used to say things like 'You poor thing' and ' Oh your poor hands 'what have you done' ' you must be in so much pain' etc. At this time my hands weren't really painful as the wrists were fused, and a couple of the middle finger joints were too but I don't think they believed me! I had to answer politely without going into detail and get them back to telling me about themselves. It did have the advantage that people realised that I would be more empathetic towards their situations, so it wasn't all bad but sometimes they felt bad for complaining about their problems!

Generally though people are not that used to working with people with disabilities, whatever disabilities you may have, and so their reactions can sometimes be over caring and pitying or they can treat you as some sort of amazing person or hero because you are out in a pub or at a concert or going on a hand glider or travelling alone on an adventurous trip or working but actually you just want to be a 'normal' person. Once my eldest daughter, who was about 20 then, was out with friends and they couldn't find a parking space and so somebody said 'We can park in this disabled space. People with disabilities don't go out in the evenings!' My daughter of course told them in no uncertain terms that they couldn't. "Her mum", she said, "often went out in the evenings" and she explained that I had a blue badge. This is typical of peoples' assumptions about disability. In her book 'The view from down here ' Lucy Webster illustrates many incidents where people made assumptions about her as she is a wheelchair user. They didn't expect her to be working or in a restaurant or out on her own or in a pub[5] "I didn't know people like you went to the pub". Although society is a bit more used to seeing people with disabilities these days than it was 25 years ago it is still not the norm to see younger people with disabilities.

During the first five years that I was working after I was qualified, I don't remember any specific RA related problems apart from opening medication bottles, the child proof ones, which I was unable to do when I was about 40 and still cannot do. Luckily, I had a husband to open them, they had to remain open but fortunately my children were older by then.

I do remember having to ask the pharmacy to open a tablet bottle on more than one occasion, but they were very reluctant to do this [or mine was anyway] as it has to be given sealed. It is a bit of a problem for people who live alone but I believe it is possible now to get non childproof tops if you specifically ask. Other than that, I had some early morning stiffness, so it has always taken me a while to get going in the morning. I just get up slowly with a tea in bed to start the day. I had to plan my day to take care that I didn't overuse a particular joint and to change

---

[5] Webster, L (2023) The View from Down here (Dorling Kingsley Ltd)

activities hourly or less whenever I could and use different joints of my body. For instance, if at home I might have done 30 minutes housework, had a coffee and sat down, walked the dog for an hour, worked on a computer for a while, done some washing up or cooked then had a sit down for a meal etc. This has become something I naturally do whenever I can.

At work as an OT, I always did a mixture of activities at a desk, talking to my patients, driving, walking around departments or people's houses to assess, going to meetings, walking to get to venues, phoning various people and so my job worked well for me. If I have to sit down for ages, I get up and walk around every now and then or go and get a drink. It's become a way of life for me. Changing positions, activities and the joints you are using is a part of joint protection and I always followed joint protection techniques as far as I could in every area of my life. There is more detail on this in the appendix.

At home I was responsible for all the cooking, I loved planning meals and trying new foods and as the kids got older, I could try new recipes.

In the kitchen I had the cooker, sink, fridge and worktops all near each other and I used lightweight pans and also, I could slide items across surfaces. I had a selection of openers, sharp knives and an L shaped bread knife with a contoured handle and I used two hands to lift the kettle.

Everyone loves my bread knife, it's easier for everyone. I used a two handled colander and a two handled large pan. I also used cutlery with coloured handles which tended to be thicker and easier to grip than metal ones and of course I still use them. The environment and your kitchen utensils are so important when you have RA. The heights of worktops, the type of controls on white goods, the type of equipment you use, having a table and chair nearby to sit and prepare food and having taps you can easily turn all make such a difference. Incidentally taps should be turned off with your left hand and on with your right so that your fingers go towards your thumb and not towards your little finger. This helps to reduce ulnar deviation. Having a kitchen environment that worked for me allowed me to carry on making meals and baking which the girls and I loved.

During this time, I still did almost all of the household chores but over the years my role has diminished although its not something that worries me too much! I used to work part time and also did pretty much all the household stuff cooking, shopping, cleaning, tidying and dusting, hoovering, ironing, changing beds and washing. This gradually become more and more difficult over the years.

In my early to mid-forties my role was reduced a bit, but I still did all the shopping, cooking, ironing, hoovering and dusting, washing floors and tidying but I became unable to manage heavy cleaning, changing beds or cleaning windows so that was delegated [what a shame!]. I also started a rota for dog walking as my time was short. I remember writing out a sheet with everything essential that I did for our household in a week itemised with the time it took. I can't recall exactly what my hours came to but something like 75! [my paid work then was about 24-30 hours a week] The extra was for dog walking, cooking, shopping, household chores, organising activities, chauffeuring teenagers around and gardening.

I was very busy during my forties and as the girls got older

Keith and I seemed to spend a lot of time driving them to places but then it became harder for me to drive my car as there was no power steering in my car then and this made parking, particularly parallel parking very difficult.

My car was always at least six years old; many small or medium cars did not have power steering before the nineties so in my mid to late forties I began to struggle a bit with the steering when there was a lot of turning involved. Also, the gears were hard for my left elbow and left knee, so I had to take care where I parked.

A little later in the nineties my oldest daughter started learning to drive which was incredibly alarming to me and very worrying as well, especially when I took her out for practise! It did mean less driving for me and Keith though and when she eventually passed her test we bought an old car for the three girls.

At this time, I was losing finger movement at the middle joints of both hands, the rotation in my wrists was very reduced as was the span of my hands. In the 1990s a tendon in my right thumb snapped and I agreed to a tendon transfer operation to replace the thumb tendon with a tendon from my fourth finger. In retrospect I probably should just have had the middle joint of the thumb fixed in a useful position because the thumb ended up fixed anyway. The tendon removed was almost certainly an extensor tendon rather than a flexor tendon that should have been used [there are 2 flexors and only 1 extensor tendon] and so the fourth finger could never extend from the middle joint any more after that operation. All these joint problems made life harder but for me it was even harder as I loved playing the clarinet and it just wasn't possible after this operation. Also, I did quite a few craft activities and these became reduced too. I was still able to drive but it became extremely difficult to get petrol. This has been tricky for me for at least 25 years and when I was working as an OT, I needed lots of petrol for visits as well as for taxiing daughters.

I have been in petrol stations, and either been unable to lift the pump or been unable to unscrew the petrol cap or both due to my reducing hand function. On more than one occasion I have been in a petrol station but there was no staff free to help me, so I had to walk up to another customer and ask them to help. The thing is when you look as if you are not disabled, and people don't always notice my hands which are the main give away, they are confused at why you are asking.

I have felt pathetic and lazy needing this help although of course no-one in this situation should feel this way. It's not as if we are lazy. The irony is it is much more hassle having to wait around for a suitable person to help than just being able to get on with the task. Anyway, on the occasions I've had to do this people have been very helpful.

At one point there was a system for petrol stations where you could let the staff know that you needed petrol, they would come out to your car. Well, that was the theory anyway, but it didn't really work as there were never many staff, the queue developed, and people wondered why staff were helping me and not taking their money at the till where there was a queue! This has not gotten any better through the years as nowadays there is often only one person serving in petrol stations.

In the mid-nineties I started to have problems with my

ankle joints, this made walking painful at times. I had some movement left in the ankles, but this is what caused pain. I would suddenly be in agony, and I was forced to stop walking for a while until it recovered. It also happened if I sat or perched, and my foot was not on the ground as on a high stool. It just seemed to dislocate. My friends got used to having to wait until the pain subsided if we were walking along the street and I had to take care getting off trains or on slopes. Downward slopes became really tricky as my ankle began to fuse, worse than uphill. I remember going to east Yorkshire and needing to go down a really steep slope in order to get on a train and having to zig zag across the slope like you do when you ski! It must have looked quite weird. I couldn't get down to visit Robin Hoods Bay at all. It was just too steep.

At the back of our garden was a gate into the farmers field and we walked the dogs over there to the lanes and countryside. It was wonderful for a couple of years and then my feet just could not cope with the uneven ground, I had to take the dog in the car to an easier, more level place. At that time as well, I was forced to stop badminton as I just could not run anymore! I had so enjoyed playing. It was such fun and great exercise for me even though I played for many years whilst having no wrist movement. My technique was to use drop shots here and there on court and at the net and catch people out but even that became impossible so sadly I had to stop playing.

The fact that I managed to keep walking three miles a day into my fifties and beyond was due to having a dog and also to podiatry and then sketchers shoes! Podiatrists treat problems with your feet such as deformities, incorrect positioning, walking and standing, as well as working as chiropodists treating bunions, dropped arches, hammer toes and nail problems.

I started attending podiatry in my forties and I had an assessment and was given orthotic insoles. As anyone knows who has had these, they are very beneficial for walking, but equally it is very difficult to fit them into ladies' shoes. They are just not deep enough. I often had to buy men's shoes in a size bigger than mine so that I could get the insoles in. Occasionally I got a women's trainer in a size bigger if there was anything suitable. I have never had a lot of choice for shoes, I have to go to a shoe shop when it is very quiet so I can try on loads of pairs. I go for comfort, never for fashion and people probably wonder why I am always in trainers but of course if it keeps you walking it's a no brainer.

As well as shoes I also started to have more restrictions with clothes. As my ankles fused, I needed trousers in bootleg style, [I couldn't and still can't get into skinny or even many straight jeans because of my lack of ankle movement!] and coupled with that I needed a shorter length and also buttons or fittings that I could open with reduced hand function. This severely reduced my choice of clothes and now it's worse.

I remember the times when I went to the shops, I had to ask for a seat in order to try trousers or shoes on. It was surprising that many shops did not have a seat available in the changing room or even in the whole shop on some occasions! Retail assistants told me that they always stood. Sometimes they went and found a footstool for me, the ones you use for putting your foot on when trying shoes, and I used that. Sometimes they lifted me a chair from another department and at other times I just had to go away and not buy anything. Now I can use online shopping and try things on at home and send them back if they don't fit. There is a parcel shop near us that's open until 10pm so that has made online shopping a little easier these days.

I also recall the time I went to the Ritz for a special treat with Keith. Often when I am planning to go out there is some organisation and planning to do first. On this occasion it involved ringing beforehand to ask the Ritz if I could come in wearing my trainers [There was a no trainer policy for visitors]. I explained that I was unable to walk without wearing trainers. Well, I could do a few steps around the house but no outside walking as my feet do not accommodate very well. Since I was 45, I've had very little or no ankle movement as my ankles have gradually over time virtually fused themselves. Once fused though they have been much less painful and stopped dislocating into extremely painful positions. Anyway, the Ritz relented, I was allowed in. I wore smart black trainers and black trousers so with a nice top it looked fine, we had a delicious cream tea. Actually, going anywhere posh like a wedding, cause me problems as my clothes have for most of my life been dictated by what I can get in and out of independently, what is comfortable and only partially by what I like to wear. Luckily, I am not and never have been crazy on fashion however I do like to have some choice.

Chapter 5: The Fourth Decade; Travel and Trauma

As I approached my fifties and my teenagers were now all 'adults' I wanted to do some more travelling. I had always loved going to new places right since I was a teenager and in my twenties. I went off hitch- hiking to Europe with friends at 18 and later on at 20 when I went to Italy, Sicily, Bavaria and Austria with a different friend. I had also enjoyed an overland camping trip to the Greek islands and in my early twenties, when Keith and I travelled in our beloved VW camper called Sammy. We drove overland to Greece and the Greek island of Aegina before there were any hotels! [we parked our van on the beach]. We also visited Denmark in our campervan and the New Forest and other UK destinations.

While we had our children with us, we often took holidays in the UK but sometimes we went further afield but those holidays were mostly beach holidays in the sun with a bit of exploring for a couple of days, but I really love to experience and explore places, sample local food and really see the local areas as well as the tourist destinations. If I could follow my heart, I would be hiking in jungles looking for gorillas or seeking out wildlife on hiking trips or visiting stunning landscapes in far flung places, but I have had to make some compromises since reaching my late forties, mostly due to my walking restrictions and to a certain degree the possibility of flare ups. That being said we have been on a few adventurous trips over the years, some were quite difficult for me due to my RA limitations.

One was particularly memorable, although it was a fantastic trip, because it was quite challenging for me at the time. I always wanted to go to Egypt to see the amazing pyramids and sphinx, the Valley of the Kings and the vast and enormous temples as well as the Cairo Museum of the pharaohs treasures. We could have gone on a more leisurely Nile cruise, but I chose to go on an Explore trip overland and on a felucca, a native Egyptian sailboat instead. It was about as adventurous as I could be with my quite severe RA.

We went via various different modes of transport, donkey, camel, felucca, coach and taxi. It was an amazing trip. The size of the temples and the pyramids and the sphynx are truly remarkable wonders but there were many tricky times for me. Sleeping on the deck of the felucca on a mattress and having to get up from the floor was very hard, as was balancing down a wooden plank to get off the boat in the night or early morning when I wanted to use the toilet! [a hole in ground with toilet seat over]. Also walking over uneven ground with feral dogs prowling about and then crouching down too were not a great experience for me!

Getting on and off a donkey was another challenge, though I wasn't too bad at staying on it once I was on! Camels presented even more difficulties. If you've ever seen these animals laboriously heaving themselves up and down, then you'll know what I mean! It's very easy to lose your balance and fall off.

I also struggled with being on a coach for seven hours as ideally you need to stretch and move every 30 mins when you have RA. Another difficult experience was being stuck tightly in a taxi when the tyre went flat, our police protection had deserted us. They continued with the other taxis who had not broken down! [This was the year after the shooting in the Valley of Kings, so we had guards with us when we travelled].

I found that 'Explore' were excellent at working with me so that I could manage to see and take part in almost everything. We also went with them to Costa Rica, which was quite adventurous too, riding a horse, trekking down to see waterfalls, white water rafting and of course jungle walks and many early morning cruises to see the spectacular bird life and enormous trees and plants. We also enjoyed sitting on the sun-drenched beaches with iguanas trying to steal our picnics!

They always explained the itinerary in detail to me before I booked, I occasionally had to miss an optional walk or had to sit something out. We did two other trips with 'Explore' and the most recent trip was Tanzania and Zanzibar. I always find that small group tours or companies that specialise in a particular country can give you a lot more information and details about a country or itinerary before you go so it's easier to make a decision. They are generally more helpful about my disability needs and restrictions too.

Incidentally my consultant was brilliant when I was going away. He gave me back up steroids for trips like this in case of a flare as with RA you cannot predict when flares will happen. These steroids got the swelling and pain under control in a day or two and I took them for two weeks then reduced them gradually every 3 or 5 days so that I took them for under 3-4 weeks in total. This avoids the risk of side effects of bone thinning that can happen when steroids are taken for longer periods or at high doses. Luckily there were no flares that I can remember on these trips. I have had them though on a west to east trip across the USA when I just had to spend a bit more time on the coach or sitting with a book or coffee somewhere. Also, I had one in Spain where I just had to have a couple of days in bed. I cannot spend my life worrying that I might have a flare or I would never go anywhere. I just book the trip and hope that I'll be ok although I must say having those steroids to hand really helped me to feel more confident that I could manage.

Unfortunately, insurance can be tricky as you become older, especially with a chronic condition, because if you want to cover all your health problems then the insurance costs far too much. These days I often choose not to cover my declared conditions. It would be unlikely that anything unplanned would happen that needed hospitalisation but of course there is always a chance, and we all have to decide about the risks we are prepared to take. The GHIC card is useful for emergency or essential health needs in the EU and other European countries and Australia though you would pay for medications, repatriations and GP visits or whatever the resident population pay for.

At this stage in my life, I had travelled to a lot of places that I had always wanted to visit. As well as the countries mentioned earlier Keith and I went to Cyprus, Portugal, Canada, Sri Lanka, New Zealand and Prague. However, there were so many more countries I wanted to see and having severe RA meant I wanted to go while I could still manage it.

Unfortunately, in 2004 our travelling was curtailed for a while. My husband Keith, our middle daughter and I were involved in a head on road traffic accident when coming back from the airport after a recent trip. The car crumpled so completely that we had to be lifted out the top and I was saved by an off-duty paramedic in a car following behind us who stopped my bleeding while we waited for help to arrive. Only the wine in the boot from Spain survived intact!

After this accident I had a few more difficulties to contend with; problems with vision in my right eye, a massive head wound, six broken ribs and a broken ankle as well as being black and blue everywhere. Keith had severe injuries to his legs and feet and a broken collarbone while our daughter had a broken collarbone too. We spent a good few months between us recovering and when we were discharged from hospital a friend had to find two wheelchairs for us from the Red Cross and that wasn't easy!

The NHS only provides wheelchairs for those with long term needs, but our injuries did not count as long term. We couldn't go home without the wheelchairs, so some friendly neighbours kindly moved our bed downstairs and found us the two temporary wheelchairs. I spent three months recovering from this and it was longer for Keith.

My OT experience was invaluable in knowing what to do and where to go for what we needed in those months. OT friends brought me a walking frame, perching stools, easy reachers, a shower attachment to wash our hair in the tiny sink in the downstairs toilet and I used my OT knowledge to help myself and my husband back to independence. I also helped Keith to get assistance from the job centre for claiming incapacity benefit as it was then, and, to start a new business as he lost his freelance engineer job immediately after the accident. The incapacity benefit was only £75 a week then so a sudden drop from his weekly full-time salary.

At times like this it is so useful to know who to speak to in order to get the things you need as quickly as possible. The NHS and Social Care can be so slow and bureaucratic when you need help and it is so frustrating when you know what you need but cannot get it and you don't know who to call and you don't know what help is available.

It is possible to get a wheelchair from the NHS, or a voucher to put towards purchasing your own, but the process is long. You have to wait for an assessment, probably weeks or months, and if you qualify it has to be ordered and this all takes time, too long for emergencies. At the time of writing the Red Cross hires wheelchairs at £22 a week and this can help out while you wait. You have to pay for delivery though or have someone to collect them. They also keep a few other essential items for the toilet, shower and walking.

Social Care can assess for care needs and provide and/or fund the care needs that are essential for everyday living. This could be homecare, adaptations, equipment, arranging personal alarms and security equipment, placements in care homes for long term care or as respite breaks for a family carer and help with placements for supported living. Even if you need to pay then you can still have advice and guidance and help with making arrangements. You will need a financial assessment to see if and how much you would need to pay. At the present time your own home is only taken in consideration for care home placements and not for home care, but this could change "Adaptations" can be funded by the council but again this depends on where you live and who owns the property. These processes are quite complicated, and the savings limit may change in the near future but if you have savings over their present limit of £23,250 then you will need to pay the full amount for homecare regardless of the financial assessment otherwise you will pay a contribution. It's also worth noting that as we both received compensation for our injuries from our insurance eventually due to the other driver being at fault, we had to pay back the incapacity benefit that Keith had claimed once we received the compensation.

When we were assessed for the compensation, we had a very incompetent consultant who produced the report. He made mistakes like which ankle was broken, and he underestimated the damage I had sustained and how long the effects were likely to last. Unfortunately, the extra complications of the crash that were triggered due to me having RA such as the flare up of my ankle after the accident couldn't be considered. His grammar and spelling were appalling and I had to send my report back three times to get it up to a reasonable standard and even then my whiplash was not considered at all. Now 20 years later I am suffering the effects in my neck and back. These effects may also be due to living with RA for 50 years.

There are excellent consultants, but you should always keep informed and check things out, especially letters, as I find there is sometimes mistakes on these and they all get transferred to our medical records that the GP holds. It is important that these records are totally accurate because they're used by health professionals, insurance companies, employers and also by Social Care.

Anyway, we got through a really difficult year, we used the compensation money in part payment for an apartment in Spain. We decided that if something bad happens like this it is a good idea to get something positive from it 'When life gives you lemons, make lemonade!'

Also, these experiences make you see that when you nearly lose your life, as I did as I had six broken ribs that only narrowly missed my lungs, as well as losing a lot of blood, then you want to go for your dreams and not waste any time. My first goal was to get my self-help book on RA published. This came to fruition in 2005, it was updated twice with the last edition being in 2011. It's taken 20 years for me to want to write another one!

Also, I wanted to raise funds and feel brave enough to talk about RA and my book on the radio on RA Awareness week and I did manage that too which made me feel very happy. Next, I wanted to continue to travel, my first goals were to go on a trip to see tigers in India and then to see giraffes and elephants in Tanzania and then to visit New Zealand and Australia. Luckily Keith is happy to travel with me. These were all amazing trips, I am so glad that I could manage to fulfil those dreams that I had had for a very long time. In a way the accident and my RA pushed me into achieving these dreams and goals. Being near to death is certainly a good motivator to live your life to the full and so I continued my passion to see more of the world.

I have found that I do have to work out well ahead how I will manage on my trips away whether it's a caravan trip in the UK or a more adventurous tour or a flight and hotel abroad. I find out as much as I can about the country I am visiting. Sometimes you have to be quite persistent to find things out but it's always worth it particularly if I am going to travel on my own which is fairly unusual for me.

Once though, I was in the Netherlands for work and the train was so high above the platform that I had to ask a stranger to lift my baggage down for me onto the platform. You cannot be shy about asking when you have RA and most people are kind and helpful. I take any equipment I might need with me, which fortunately isn't usually much, but I find my own knife and scissors useful. Once I forgot to put the knife into my hold baggage and the x-rays picked it up in my hand luggage so that disappeared for good! I also take snacks to take with anti-inflammatory tablets, and I always make a list a few days before I go to ensure I don't forget anything vital like having plenty of medication in case of delays or emergencies. We have had one or two of those like being trapped by volcanic ash in Spain.

Three months after the accident. I returned to work. I wanted to change from my usual assessment work. Before the accident I was working on an enablement project which was being set up to allow Social Care clients to have care that was enabling rather than having care that was given to them. After the accident I went back to assessing people in their homes, but this could sometimes be challenging for me.

Whilst visiting clients I could never be quite sure what the environment would be like when I arrived. As an OT my remit was wide. I was helping to enable my clients to be as independent as possible in daily activities, personal care, leisure, work, education and getting about. Sometimes I needed to take measurements for an extension, a stairlift or for a wheelchair or in the bathroom for level access showers. I often had to go into every room to assess, I had to set up equipment ready for people to try. The property could be level access or there could be 30 steps to a flat with no lift! The doors could be tricky to open or the stairs in some houses, particularly Victorian ones, could be ultra steep and narrow with no rails. Opening tricky doors to get outside into the garden or needing to fight my way through endless clutter with barely any space to walk through was a challenge too. The difficulties were becoming more and more of a problem but one thing that made my working life more difficult did get sorted out and that was the parking.

I needed to park as close as I could to the clients, because of having to carry equipment, but up to that time I did not have severe enough difficulties for obtaining a blue badge and I did not claim any disability benefits. I had never really needed to, and I wouldn't have qualified anyway.

My OT manager explained that I should apply for a blue badge as it would enable me to keep working. She also said to apply for DLA as this would help me to pay for extra things that I needed to pay out for as a disabled person. I did need to purchase aids sometimes, like my bath lift, and parking was needed for longer as it took me more time to get anywhere. Also, I had to pay for my medications because having a chronic condition did not mean that I got them free. Thinking about these things allowed me to feel I was justified, I applied for both and was successful for both. Up to this time I hadn't really thought of myself as a disabled person. I'd always done my best to find solutions to any problem that came along, although it's true that it may well be hard for many people with RA to work full time and this inevitably means a lower income. Fortunately, I was mostly able to work part time after I had children and this meant work was more manageable for me, but many people will need two full time incomes nowadays just to live.

Blue badges are given to people who have extreme difficulty in moving around even for short distances, often due to severe pain, fatigue or breathlessness, sensory difficulties or mental health problems like anxiety. The blue badge means you can park closer to where you need to go. You can be awarded a badge at any age, you don't need to drive to receive it. If you receive the highest mobility component of DLA or some categories of PIP, which has replaced DLA, you will be awarded a blue badge automatically.

Having disabilities in both of your arms and hands may also qualify you for a blue badge if you drive. Personal Independence Payment [PIP] is awarded to anyone over 16 and under pension age who has a substantial and long-term disability [physical or mental health] which has an impact on their everyday life. It is not means tested and is awarded to help disabled people manage their extra living costs.

Both the blue badge and the DLA were enormously helpful and did help me to stay working, but carrying things and setting them up was still a problem as my hand function got worse as did my mobility on uneven ground and steep stairs. Due to these issues during my last years of employment I worked on a Carers and Work project for two years then came back to working as an OT, but it was during this time that I nearly ended up losing my job. At this point I was in my mid-fifties and certainly did not want to stop yet and couldn't afford to either.

One day I made the mistake of telling my manager that one of these days I would get trapped inside someone's house and not be able to open the door to leave. This was said as a joke. I never thought it would really happen but occasionally my clients had had to let me out of their house! My manager was worried that if someone became aggressive, I would not be able to leave and at this time we did not have work mobiles and we worked alone [It's possible that I had my own basic phone I can't recall for certain]. Anyway, a meeting was set up with the HR representative and I had to have a health and safety assessment. Then there was another meeting where the District Manager suddenly appeared and told me out of the blue that I would have to leave if I couldn't find an alternative job in the council in the next three months!

I was devastated and promptly burst into tears. It was so sudden, and if I did find a job the salary would be much lower, and I still had about five years to go to 60 which was the retirement date for women at that time. I had a quick look on the council website but anything I saw was at a much lower salary and a lot less interesting. Also, the council bases your pension on the last three to five years you are working so my pension would be lowered too.

While I was mulling this over, I had a sudden thought. I had just remembered that there was a Disability Discrimination Act and that I should have been allowed reasonable adjustments to keep working and this had not even been suggested at the meeting. I promptly wrote a clear and concise letter to my manager outlining what the department could do to help and why he should support me with this and stating that I had not been offered any 'reasonable adjustments' yet. This produced a complete turnaround, and positions were found for me that I could manage safely, mainly in the office. I did referral management, supporting the team taking referrals and helping the OT assistants. I then applied and was accepted for a one-year position supporting staff with the new databases that were now in use and then I started assessing people in care homes. After this somehow no-one seemed to mind when I was asked to help out with assessing people in the community again!

Perhaps this was because the department had brought in Access to Work who said that I needed someone to support me on visits as well as the option of working from home for completing my admin tasks, but somehow an assistant to accompany me did not materialise as it cost money! [The employer has to pay towards the costs and then Access to Work provide the rest]. I was given a computer system which I could use while I was at home on my own PC which was a help, but otherwise I assessed clients over the phone and worked out whether I could do the visit. If I thought, it would be difficult then I passed it to someone else or got an OT assistant to go with me. I therefore managed to hold onto my job until I decided to take redundancy at 60 when the council decided it couldn't afford many OTs and SWs that year due to budget cuts!

The pension age was 61 years and 5 months for me by that time, but I was happy that I was able to work until 60 as many people with disabilities struggle both to get work and even more to stay in work. According to government statistics [6] 53.1% of disabled people were employed compared to 81.6% for non-disabled people in 2024.

I definitely think that a suitable job that you enjoy gives lots of benefits mentally and physically. You have more money and make friends; you have a useful role in society and for me helping people with disabilities to improve the quality of their life was something I loved and worked hard at. If I had any stress, pain or trauma going on in my personal life then work helped me to focus on something else and gave me a reason to get up when I had a lot of pain and stiffness.

During my fifties I did have some flare ups. I had been on Sulphasalazine for many years and at that point I don't think it was really controlling my RA enough. I was still getting more and more joint damage. My ankles became virtually fused, a couple of toes became fused, the span of my hand reduced and my fingers were getting worse. I could still walk for a couple of miles though, when I wasn't in a flare up, but things were getting worse. When I asked for different medication, I was tried on Hydrochloroquine. I had to stop taking it when my eyes started to be damaged although they were back to normal once I stopped it.

I then tried Leflunomide but it caused unexplained bruising, and I could not have Methotrexate as it was likely to cause nodules, on my fingers which I already tended to get a lot.

---

[6] Official Statistics (2025) The Employment of Disabled People 2024 gov.uk/the employment of disabled people

At this point I really needed to have the newer biologic treatments.

Biologics were first approved for RA in 1998 when I was 47 but they were not really used much for RA until the first decade of the 21st century when I was in my early fifties. I asked about them in my late fifties, but I was initially told that I did not qualify for them as my disease activity score, known as DAS was not high enough.

At that time, I found out how DAS scores are measured from NRAS [7]. I didn't know much about them before that although they started being used to measure disease activity in the 1990's in some areas. DAS stands for disease activity score. Your disease activity score is given to you by your consultant who observes how many joints in your body are hot, swollen or inflamed. He also considers your scores for erythrocyte sedimentation score[esr] and c-reactive protein [CRP] from your blood tests as these are inflammatory markers. [you need these levels checked regularly when you are taking DMARDS].

The consultant should also check the patient's own views about their joints and then arrive at a score. It needs to be at least 3.2 for you to be given biologics. Nowadays you can have an app on your phone to measure your DAS score. For more information about DAS have a look at the NRAS publication New2RA.

This process did not work well for me because my RA does

---

[7] The DAS 28 score (2025) nras.org/resource

not often cause complete flare ups affecting my whole body, but more often I have had flares of particular joints and sometimes the damage just gets gradually worse but with no bells and whistles to announce it at all, just stiffness and discomfort. This has probably been lucky for me in many ways but in other ways it means damage is occurring continually and it's difficult for me to prove it except by scans and x-rays but by then the damage has already been done!

Also, for some inexplicable reason the joints of the feet and ankles do not contribute to the number of flared joints you have when your DAS is assessed. I was told it is because feet are problematic in OA as well, so they don't count! Thirdly you don't often have an appointment during a flare and even if you try to get one then the joint has often settled by then or in my case, I had taken a short steroid course to knock it out. I didn't really want to wait in agony with reduced abilities and no end of pain and damage being done just to get the joint counted in a DAS score! As I wasn't able to qualify this meant I took too much Ibuprofen as it was the only thing that magically reduced my pain, stiffness and inflammation and got me moving. The Ibuprofen eventually caught up with me later on though but at the time it was the only thing that kept me moving and living my life.

Around this time, at the end of my working life, I was very lucky to have an opportunity to travel to Barcelona with NRAS. I had entered 'my story' for a chance to be one of a few representative members of NRAS to go and tell their story for a celebration 'My day for RA' I was really happy to be selected. I think my story is still on the NRAS website! My husband went with me as my carer, and we had a wonderful time. I could visit many of the sites by the tourist bus, walk down the Ramblas from our hotel, use the wonderful swimming pools in the hotel and we all contributed to sharing our stories.

There were people with RA from all over Europe and we could swap stories and ideas, and we were filmed together. During this celebration of NRAS we were presented with a special book of poems from the actress Jane Seymour. It was a very special day, I was so glad that I had entered! NRAS is such a brilliant organisation. You can learn so much from their information and their self-management modules, you can become involved in fundraising and RA Awareness week and there are local groups and online presentations too. In fact, there is so much volunteering needed in the UK that you can continue to work as long as you want but of course you won't get paid! In the next chapter I will cover my life with RA as a retired person who volunteers!

Chapter 6: The Fifth Decade; Life after Work

During the last three years or so that I was working I began to think about what I could do when I retired. I wanted to work but, I had to be realistic about what I could manage as I got older, with the RA progressing and my joints still deteriorating. I thought about working in the area of employment as an OT, but it turned out that there were not that many openings in this field and I needed a job in my local area. I interviewed for about three jobs but I did not have the experience to get any of the jobs on offer, so I thought about training as a life coach.

I had done a basic course two or three years back and I thought that life coaching would be just right for me to do part time. Life coaching has lots of similarities to O.T. except you work with anyone who feels stuck in their life not just people with disabilities. It's about helping people to work out what they want to do and then coaching them to plan to achieve their goals. Even better, I did not need to be physically able as long as I could drive and walk a little. And in fact, I could have set up in my own home if need be. Firstly, I chose a course to complete. I had to do a long weekend intensive course and then I worked with some volunteer clients for a few months while I was studying and writing assignments to pass the course.

The weekend course was a bit of a hurdle. The first night before the course started, I booked into a bed and breakfast nearby. On arriving with my very light case on wheels that I thought I could manage independently I realised that I had to somehow lift this case up a spiralling staircase to get to my room! On the reception was a very old man who looked like he would have more difficulty than me so I didn't feel I could ask him for assistance! I did manage to reach my room somehow! The next day I was booked into a grand looking hotel, but it was a really, really old building. I struggled to open all the doors to get in and out of my room or any room in the building come to that. The doors were so heavy with large round handles, just the type I can never turn. Since then, I have been a lot more careful when booking rooms, however, once on the course many people turned out to be very helpful. It’s important to be honest and to have the confidence to ask for help when it’s needed.

Once trained I worked with an organisation called Life Clubs, setting up small local groups to help people make positive changes in their lives, then, after this I decided to go freelance and set up my own business with my own clients. This was very rewarding; I could work at home or in a local venue or at a client’s home and the times of sessions were arranged to suit us both. I did not need many physical abilities for this work, and I only needed to do a few hours a week, so it worked very well for me. I do remember though the days when I really struggled to get up, out and drive to my client’s house but I didn’t want to let people down so I hardly ever cancelled.

Life coaching can be incredibly helpful for anyone who is feeling stuck and unable to work out the way ahead. It can help with employment, family life and relationships, diet, gaining confidence and any aspect of life where change is needed. It's about learning to look at things in different ways and believing in yourself and understanding how to set realistic goals. You learn about yourself, find out what you want to do, and then plan a course of action to achieve your goals. It can be very useful for people with RA who often have to accept a new reality on many occasions and then need to find different or flexible and creative ways to move forward.

I really loved helping people, I find that if I am really engaged and passionate about what I am doing then the pain and stiffness is less noticeable as my focus is elsewhere [unless I am in really acute pain]. Seeing and hearing about other peoples' problems allows you to escape your own for a while!

I do have to be careful and organised and think ahead at all times because of the difficulties I have had for many years due to my very reduced hand function. For instance, I have to be very careful not to drop my keys when I'm out by myself, if they go down in the middle of the car or under a seat or if they roll under the car I cannot get them back. I can recall this happening a few times over the years. Once I was parked in an underground carpark under our OT office. I accidentally dropped the keys; they became wedged in a place where I could not pull them out due to not being able to slip my fingers into the space. Anyone else could have got them out quite easily. Things like this can potentially be a problem for me though because my fingers are fused at the middle joints and so my fingers don't straighten, they often won't fit into gaps. There was no one around to ask and so I had to walk back up to my office and find a helpful work colleague to come and assist. It wasn't that much of a problem for them, but it did hold them up and we were always incredibly busy. These incidents make you feel as if you are being a nuisance and although it has got easier to ask over the years it is none the less slightly embarrassing and people do not always understand why you can't do things yourself.

I did the life coaching for about six years but even when I stopped, when I was around 65, I always loved to be making a difference or helping out with things, although I have to take care when choosing activities. The first volunteer role I had when I left OT was as a dog walker for the Cinnamon trust and also, I did a little dog fostering too. I had to choose the dogs carefully as I needed them to be well trained and not too strong. I have always loved dogs; I had always walked our own dogs every day. In my early 60's I could still manage this although I did walk later in the day as it always takes me a while to get going due to stiffness and my natural disposition towards being a night owl rather than a lark. You can also walk for local kennels or sign up to borrowmydoggy.com! It's great for exercise if you like dogs.

It is important to exercise as much as you can when you have RA. You need to keep your muscles strong to support weakened joints and you need to maintain your range of movements at each joint as much as possible. Also exercise helps to control cholesterol and osteoporosis as well as helping to reduce blood pressure. It's important to keep within your own limits though and it's better to do a few short sessions daily or weekly rather than go mad on one day. This applies to domestic chores, cooking, shopping, gardening or anything physical. Exercise can be any physical activity that you love and can manage without incurring lots of pain. You don't need to go to a gym or hike or run or do classes. You can dance or play table tennis or do any sport you love; you could swim or hula hoop or work in the garden or do yoga. Anything that is using muscles and working your heart a little. Maybe a mini trampoline or skipping or playing golf. Just do what you fancy and if you can get someone to join you all the better. Even a short walk for a coffee can be beneficial. There are health walks you can join too and these are graded and different lengths. The local council website has details, and you can just turn up to join in. These are run during the weekdays though, so they are only useful for retired or unemployed people or those who work flexibly from home.

There are three types of exercise we all need, firstly those for strengthening muscles -Tai Chi is good for this. Secondly aerobic exercise to improve the cardiovascular system and maintain a healthy weight. Anything that speeds your heart up is aerobic exercise. Lastly you should also try to incorporate range of movement exercise. This means putting all your joints through their natural range of movements every day. If this does not happen naturally then it's a good idea to build some exercises into your day.

On the NRAS website there are videos on getting started and basic exercises and Tai Chi too. Remember exercise is very important and it should not be forgotten even if it can feel like the last thing you want to do. Having said that take care in a flare or if a particular joint is causing you pain. Sometimes I feel very angry that I love to exercise and would happily play sports or go for long walks while so many people who are able to do this just don't want to walk even a few metres. These are the people who park very close to venues and then there are no spaces for those people who need to be near but don't quite qualify for a blue badge.

I was originally as a child and teenager very sporty and full of energy. In my twenties I walked for miles and played tennis and rode a bike. I also loved gardening. Things got harder once I had RA but we had dogs for about 30 years and they are great for getting you out of the house in all weathers. I always walked three miles a day when I had a dog although I did have to restrict myself to smoother, less bumpy surfaces and wear supportive shoes to do it after I was in my late forties. I also swam regularly, and this is an activity many people will be able to manage, it exercises lots of different joints and raises your heartbeat too. Then there was gardening and dancing. Lately I have been doing exercises to my Spotify playlist!

As well as maintaining strength, exercise also promotes wellbeing by raising serotonin levels and this makes us feel happier. Walking in nature is also good for our mental health. If you can exercise with a friend there are added benefits too, because after all if someone else is involved, you are more likely to keep the exercise up as you support each other and enjoy each other's company.

You could also try Pilates or yoga or anything you fancy as long as you have some of each type of exercise. Thirty minutes a day is all you need and regular daily exercise is better than loads at the weekend. Even if you cannot do a lot get up from your chair every 30 minutes and move around; make a drink, make the bed, walk round the garden, do a few exercises or go up and down some stairs. You can exercise on a chair, on the bed, standing or at a table. Just build it into your routine so it becomes second nature. Now that many people work from home, at least on some days, it may be easier to build in some exercise.

It is worth noting that the NHS presently has an exercise referral scheme [8] for people over 16 who are exercising less than thirty minutes a week and at moderate risk of developing a long-term health condition like diabetes, cardio-vascular conditions, osteoporosis and mental health conditions. This could be helpful for some people with RA. It also shows that the NHS is recognising that it's better for your health to keep active in any way that you can because of the benefits to health.

I also volunteered as a meet and greet representative for the Wildlife trust. I loved this as it involved talking to visitors about the birds, plants and trees on our reserve and the role of the British Wildlife trusts. Also selling beautiful gifts from our shop. I was in my mid to late sixties then with restricted walking and standing and some things were tricky for me. However, most things were possible, even if I had to scoop out coins from the till with a teaspoon or ask someone to turn the tap on for me when I wanted a coffee! I loved my role there and I volunteered until there was a change in my job role during covid, when it involved being outside for long stints, and I hate being in the cold and rain!

---

[8] The NHS Gym/Exercise Referral scheme (2025) the fitnessgrp.co.uk/nhs-gp-exercise-referral-scheme

Mostly, I find people are quite helpful and accommodating, and so many volunteers are needed these days that there will always be something interesting to do. Leaving the wildlife trust meant I could start somewhere else when the opportunity presented itself, however, in 2019 I had had a massive deterioration in my physical health, it was not the best timing as covid soon followed! I did learn a lot about hospitals, referrals and project managing my various NHS journeys though, as well as learning how to manage excruciating pain and cope with many frustrations while still trying my best to keep myself strong, positive and determined!

At the end of May 2019 my left knee flared and blew up like a balloon. I had been waiting to get a new biologic medication, but I never seemed to have a high enough disease activity score to achieve it. My consultant was sympathetic, and she realised how badly I needed it, and so at this time with this flare up and a few other dodgy joints I qualified at last which was brilliant. There was a downside though as my rheumatologist wanted to wait for the medication to kick in before referring me to the orthopaedic specialist for a knee replacement.

In the middle of June, I suddenly had severe back pain and excruciating sciatica pain burning down my right leg. Both of these made it impossible to walk even one step without extreme pain. Getting out of bed in the early morning was the worst and I had to use all my willpower to get out of bed and get to the bathroom. My new medication did not start until August 2019 and in the end, it was September before I was referred to the orthopaedic consultant. At this time my x-rays showed almost no cartilage around my knee joint.

Meanwhile I was wrestling with everyday practicalities and trying to help to improve my situation while I waited. This involved many frustrating calls and visits to the GP as I requested equipment to help me to walk in the house. Luckily, I still had my mum's NHS wheelchair so that helped. No-one at the GP practice seemed to know who to refer to for walking frames. I was contacted firstly by an OT, then a district nurse, before finally a community physio called me. It took a couple of weeks to get the gutter [elbow] frame and two walking sticks that were suitable for me.

I found a private physiotherapist in relation to my back issues as I wanted to keep my muscles as strong as I could before my replacement knee operation, but this was extremely difficult with so much pain. Later on, I went to an NHS physiotherapist and struggled onto the sessions on two sticks. I tried to keep up social contacts, friends and family as well because seeing people did help to take the focus off the pain, although it was difficult to even get comfortable in a chair at this time because of the intense sciatica pain.

I remember going to our local independent cinema which has luxurious seats and level access entry, but even then, I had to periodically stand up to change position and relieve the pain a bit; no doubt annoying all the people behind me!

My husband and I had booked a river cruise on the Rhine, and I couldn't decide what to do about it as we had paid in full by this time. Eventually we decided that I would give it a go despite the pain and practical difficulties [We would have lost all the money otherwise]. I telephoned to let the company know the situation and although they were trying to help, they asked reams of questions about my wheelchair. Eventually they concluded that I could bring it onto the boat but not into my cabin! So, then I asked if I could bring a walking frame into our cabin, [as I could not walk without it] I was told it might be too wide, and they needed measurements. I responded that it was the same width as me and that there would probably be a few people larger than me on the boat [who presumably didn't give their measurements!] Anyway, finally the walking frame was allowed on!

The trip went pretty well apart from the weather but what I had not realised was that the floor I had chosen for our cabin which was central for getting to the dining area and to walk on/off the boat was not always level with the land when we moored! Many times, it was, but three or four times we had to walk onto the shore from the highest deck and that was murder for me! I had to climb up no end of steps with only a rope to hold onto to disembark and then down the steps again when we returned. It was incredibly painful. However, it was lovely watching the world going by from my bed in the cabin and the meals were to die for. Actually, the tour guides were great at going through the next day's excursions and we worked out how and if I could manage them. Once I was home, I started my new RA medication at last.

Eventually, after I had waited four months in agony on the waiting list for my knee operation, I called and asked for a cancellation. I had been on the cancellation list, but nothing had been offered. By this time, I had had to buy a raised toilet seat as well and use Codeine to sleep due to the intense pain on both sides of my body. This time when I rang, I was asked did I mind changing consultants and could I come in in six days' time! Of course, I said I would go anywhere at any time with any consultant who could perform a total knee replacement operation! Then they said, 'shouldn't you stop your immunosuppressants two weeks before?' I promptly replied that my consultant said I could take a cancellation and just stop the immunosuppressant medication as soon as I could. [At least I think she said that, and I am sure she would have agreed!] I had my operation on leap year day 2020 only ten days before everything shut down for covid. I was so lucky!

The new knee was amazing, I was asked if I wanted pain medication so many times and I instantly responded that whatever small amount of pain I had now it was nothing to what I had experienced before the operation. I was out of hospital two days later and by using masses of ice to bring down the swelling and following all the exercises each day my knee was good as new in a few weeks. It was brilliant.

I now had to deal with the sciatica. I had hoped that this would go once the knee operation was done but unfortunately this did not happen, I was really disappointed that I could not get back to the two mile walks I could do in 2019. I was exercising but it did not help and then in the autumn 2020 I had another health problem. I had to have investigations, and it turned out that I had an ulcer in my oesophagus and a hiatus hernia which was causing some problems with heartburn. This was most probably due to the continual Nurofen that I have needed to take since I was 40 to control stiffness and allow me to move. It has been a life saver but of course all medications have their downsides and sooner or later this was going to catch up with me. Of course, since then I have had to take proton pump inhibitors or PPIs like omeprazole which may also cause side effects especially if taken continually.

In relation to the sciatica nerve pain, I've tried various medications that I have been offered such as Gabapentin and Amitriptyline I've also tried Dihydrocodeine and Codeine, which are opioid pain killers and become addictive if taken for long. Lastly, I've taken Paracetamol, a simple analgesic and Naproxen, an anti-inflammatory medication. None of these made any difference at all to the sciatica that I have been experiencing and almost all of these cause problems when taken long term, though they may be useful for some people for short term pain.

The only thing that helps me to some extent is the Nurofen [Ibuprofen] that has unfortunately been causing me gastric problems. I have chosen to reduce it to one slow release capsule a day, a compromise.

Recently I attended a pain management appointment and the consultant emphasised the need to take a biopsychosocial approach to the sciatica pain. That is, to use a variety of modes like Paracetamol along with low impact exercises for the back to strengthen the core muscles. Also, a TENS machine was suggested, as well as hot and cold compresses, massage and the use of a topical gel like Voltarol. To this I personally would add doing any activities you enjoy that can be managed with the pain, social interactions, a chat over coffee or lunch with friends and/or family or immersing yourself into a book, podcast or film. Choose whatever you love to do [as long as it's legal!]

I did have some success with the TENS machine as it reduced the sciatica significantly for two or three years but now it does not seem to help me anymore. I have always done back exercises every day for the last five years and although it does not remove the pain it does help me to stay mobile. I have used hot and cold applications for inflammation and swelling that have proved useful. I have found massage does relieve tension and is relaxing and this can help to reduce pain levels but it's very expensive as is acupuncture which I have also tried. Unfortunately, it didn't work for me, I had six sessions, but it can be helpful for some people.

An international research collaboration, involving the University of York, has shown that acupuncture is an effective treatment for chronic pain in patients with chronic back and neck pain, osteoarthritis, shoulder pain, and chronic headache.[9] 17,922 participants were enrolled in 29 high quality, randomized trials. The trials took place over a number of years and the study measured how well acupuncture relieved chronic pain associated with these four pain conditions.

I was also offered a steroid injection into my spine, but it has not reduced my pain but apparently it works well for some people. Lastly, I have tried medicinal cannabis and Voltarol gel but unfortunately with no success. I am now exploring the surgical options. I am determined to reduce this debilitating sciatica and back pain and increase my walking and standing

[9] MacPherson, Dr H *et al* (2017) Acupuncture is of benefit to some types of chronic pain york.ac.uk

tolerance.

As I have always hated taking medications and I have over the years explored many supplementary or alternative treatments. I tried an elimination diet but did not find any food that was causing me problems. I have had hypnotherapy and healing and homeopathy and reflexology. I have also tried various supplements. I did a lot of research into complementary treatments for my earlier book [last edition in 2011] but I could only find benefits in relation to eating a Mediterranean diet. This diet advises eating lots of fruit and vegetables, whole grains, olive oil and fish, particularly oily fish, which is rich in omega 3 oils. These can help to reduce inflammation and improve stiffness.[10] Research has shown that following a mediterranean diet can improve symptoms of RA. This included reduced swollen and tender joints and duration of morning stiffness. General wellbeing was also seen to improve.

I have researched again whilst writing this book but very little has really changed in relation to diet, supplements or complementary therapies. Ginger has been shown to have anti-inflammatory benefits; it also improves circulation for people with Raynaud's phenomenon.

I did find the following article promoting a plant-based diet and this may help to reduce the inflammatory effects like pain and swelling.[11] The article noted that 'Several studies have

---

[10] Benefits of the Mediterranean anti-inflammatory diet, (2025) nras.org/resource/diet

[11] Nutrition Interventions in Rheumatoid Arthritis: The Potential Use of Plant-Based Diets. A Review, (2019)

shown that joint pain and other RA symptoms may be modified by dietary factors. Excessive body weight and diets that include animal products (e.g., dairy, red meat) exacerbate the RA symptoms, likely due to their pro-inflammatory effects. In contrast, diets rich in vegetables, fruits and fibre are associated with lower BMI, have anti-inflammatory properties and help reduce pain and inflammation in these patients' This is definitely worth bearing in mind. I do eat lots of vegetables, fruit and fibre and I have reduced my intake of pro-inflammatory foods like red meat, dairy, processed foods and sugary foods. I don't want to take them out totally as it's good to eat a little of the food you love. Fortunately, I really like fruit, vegetables and salads too!

In relation to everyday food intake vitamin D, calcium and iron are especially important for people with RA because we are more at risk of becoming low in iron and also more likely to have osteoporosis. Therefore, anyone with RA needs to ensure that their intake of vitamin D is sufficient as it is needed to process calcium. Of course there is very little sunshine in the UK, even in summer, so we cannot maintain vitamin D levels in our bodies to last all the year and that's another reason for vitamin D supplements.

Of course, it is important that everyone gets enough calcium in their diet as well, to ensure that their bones stay strong and healthy. This is an even greater consideration when you have RA; especially if you are using steroids as part of your

---

https://www.frontiersin.org/journals/nutrition/articles/10.3389/fnut.2019.00141/full

treatment, as this may put you at a higher risk of developing osteoporosis.

Iron is a mineral that's needed because it is a vital component of haemoglobin, a component of our red blood cells, that transport oxygen from the lungs to all the parts of the body and the muscles. Iron is also needed to prevent anaemia, a deficiency of red blood cells, making it harder to transport oxygen around the body. Anaemia can be caused by chronic inflammation, medications and impaired iron absorption. Therefore, adequate dietary intake of iron is important to help prevent fatigue. Iron is more easily absorbed by the body if you have it at the same time as vitamin C, so have a portion of fruit or a small glass of fruit juice with your meals. There is a very good article on rheumatoid arthritis and diet on the BDA website.[12]

In summary[13] Diet won't cure rheumatoid arthritis (RA), but the right food choices can help by controlling the inflammation that wreaks havoc in the body, delivering nutrients your body needs and helping you maintain a healthy weight. That's important because excess weight adds to pressure on achy joints and can make certain RA meds less effective. What's more, body fat produces proteins called cytokines that promote inflammation.

We can see that it's important to eat lots of fruit and vegetables, also to include wholegrain foods including

---

[12] Rheumatoid Arthritis and Diet (2025) factsheet, bda.uk.com

[13] Best foods for Rheumatoid Arthritis (2025) Arthritis Foundation arthritis.org

wholemeal bread, rice and pasta, beans and pulses for fibre, healthy unsaturated fats like oily fish with omega 3 oils, nuts and seeds and also some protein in lean meat, fish, eggs and tofu. Foods to avoid or eat less of are saturated fats, processed foods, red meat, sugary drinks including too many fruit juices, confectionary and white food products as these make inflammation more likely.

As I have got older, I have found that the number of medical appointments that I need and the difficulty that I have balancing medications has increased. As I stated earlier less exercise can mean more likelihood of osteoporosis and high cholesterol, diabetes and cardiac problems.

Taking medications also means more side effects which may bring you other problems. For instance, in my case the RA medication Baricitinib can mean higher cholesterol but it's great for controlling RA, Nurofen means possible gastric problems, but it helps me to move more easily. One of the medications I take to lower blood pressure can cause swollen ankles or affect your kidneys. Omeprazole to protect the stomach may have short term effects on your stomach e.g. flatulence or constipation. Long term it can reduce magnesium levels which can cause various things including tiredness and dizziness and B12 deficiency. This then affects iron levels and so can lead to tiredness and mouth ulcers and also bone fractures.

This means that when you are taking medications for RA and associated health problems you must ensure that you have three monthly blood checks so that these problems can be picked up. Your rheumatologist and your GP will set these tests up for you but make sure that they are not forgotten and look at your results. You may be able to view them online or ask for a print off if you do not have online access.

In this day and age of digital recording you might expect that GPs and consultants can see the results of blood tests but that is not necessarily the case. My rheumatologist cannot see my blood test results and has to request them from the GP. Same with scans of all types. They can only be shared if requested. I attend five different hospitals and there is little shared information except sometimes letters to my GP and these often take a long time to arrive. These hospitals are all in different health areas so you can never make assumptions about what is going on and what will happen. Always check things out and follow them up. You are probably the only one who knows what's going on in each different health or community service and you are definitely the main expert on your own body. This is why project management is so important!

Chapter 7: Some Positive Changes for RA 1974-2024

I am now into my sixth decade with RA and this will probably be my hardest due to the damage to most of my joints as well as my spine. In the last year alone, I have had two operations, I probably need one or two more. One good thing that has happened recently though is my Motability car.

I have received DLA mobility payments for quite a few years now, but I have never used them to lease a new car under the Motability scheme before. I used to save the money and fund any disability needs that I had, including saving for a second-hand car. I now have a Motability car which is electric and of course automatic and it's brilliant.

I can charge it on my drive, it gets taken for services regularly at no cost to me. It has free breakdown included and it is so easy to drive. I don't need to worry if it goes wrong as I get a replacement and I can have a new one every three years!

Driving is absolutely crucial for my independence, now that my walking is limited to about five minutes on a good day, so it's wonderful for me and anyone else who struggles to walk.

Another positive thing to note is that my RA is now well under control, I have had almost no flares since I started taking Baricitinib. I do, however, have a whole range of medical issues at the moment and rather than focus on those in this last chapter I want to focus on the future for people with RA now. Things are so much more positive nowadays than they were for me when my RA started.

Anyone who is diagnosed now or in recent years will probably be able to carry on their life with very few changes once their medication controls their inflammation and slows down their disease or brings remission. Since the seventies the choice of safe and efficient DMARD medications have grown extensively.

As I said in chapter 3 the only DMARDS that I could have been offered in the 70s and 80s were Sulphasalazine and Methotrexate and also gold therapy which was used a lot in the seventies.

Interestingly I found this excerpt from a study in Canada reviewed by Paul Davis[14] which said 'For many years, gold therapy has been the mainstay in the management of patients with progressive rheumatoid disease. At the present time two forms of gold therapy are available: one by injection and the other by the oral route. A significant number of patients will achieve clinical benefit from treatment with one of these two compounds. Both compounds have a high prevalence of side-effects and should be regarded as toxic, although the oral preparation appears to have a somewhat better safety profile than has the injectable compound.'

I can remember people saying that they were being treated with gold therapy here in the UK when I first went to

[14] Davis, P; (1998) Gold Therapy in the Treatment of Rheumatoid Arthritis Feb;34:445, 447, 449, 451- [452].

rheumatology although thankfully, I was not offered it!

The next DMARD that became available was Hydroxychloroquine which was first used for malaria and then found to be beneficial for RA in the 1990s. Lastly Leflunomide, which I also tried, was developed for RA and found to be effective and safe around the late 1990s. All these conventional DMARDS work effectively, at least for many people with RA, sometimes in combination but they tend to dampen down many aspects of the immune system as they are not targeted.

Fortunately, breakthroughs in science in the early years of the twentieth century have led to a better understanding of what happens within the immune system in people with RA, while protein engineering has led to the possibility of selectively inhibiting harmful cells that are causing RA.

These new selective drugs are called the Biologic drugs [Biologic means they are made from proteins from living cells]. The biologic medicines are given by injections or infusions. There are many different types now and some work better on some people than others and so sometimes it can take a while to find the best one for each individual. Peoples' reactions to drugs and side effects vary but there is now plenty of choice so usually remission or low activity can be achieved for almost everyone with RA.

There are also biosimilars now which started to be made by different manufacturers once the originator drugs were at the end of their patent. These are not identical, but they have to be as safe and effective as the originators and there are rigid standards to comply with. Some people on the original biologics are being gradually changed onto the biosimilars as these are a lot less costly.

Since around 2017 a new class of drugs has been developed, these are the JAK Inhibitors. They are also targeted but they can be taken in tablet form because they are small-molecules therapies that work inside the cell while biologics are large-molecule therapies that work by blocking action on the outside of cells [and because they are large, they can't be taken orally]. These new JAK Inhibitors are effective and have a safe profile, but they will now not be offered to people over 65 or those at risk of cardiovascular disease or cancer as a precaution.

I take these and they do work very well for me. I have been on them since 2019 and have had no problems with my RA since then and I was over 65 when I started on them, but these risk factors were not known originally, only the short-term side effects. I have found that my cholesterol has been a bit higher since I started them but it could be because I have been far less active since 2019.

It has to be said though that when you are first diagnosed you will be started on the conventional DMARDS and will only be offered the biologics if the conventional DMARDS are not effective or cause problematic side effects. Later on, if you start having more flare ups showing that the medication is losing effectiveness you could then be considered for newer medications. The National Institute for Health and Care Excellence NICE [15] has guidelines which say you must have tried at least two conventional DMARDs used in combination

[15] Rheumatoid arthritis in adults: management (2025) nice.org.uk/guidance

[usually including Methotrexate] and if these have not been effective or the side effects cannot be tolerated then you can be considered for Biologics or JAK inhibitors if they are appropriate. You must also have high levels of disease activity as measured by DAS, 3.2-5.1 [see earlier section on DAS.]

Medication has vastly improved since the 70s when my disease started but what else has improved for people diagnosed with RA now?

As an older person with RA myself and because I did not get a diagnosis until far too late in the day, I now have extensive joint damage. Nowadays the diagnosis should be much quicker. Also, there is much more availability of various types of scans around now than when I was young, which is really helpful too. I don't think anyone realised quite how much damage I had in my joints. These days it would be picked up much more quickly and also the available surgery would be more successful and beneficial if it should be needed.

Replacing the joints in your fingers, shoulders, elbows, knees or hips will have much better results, especially as the replacements are lighter and last for longer. Ironically, there is greater skill in surgery for RA now, but it's less often needed. Indeed, on the NRAS website [16] it states that "Surgery, like all areas of medicine, is improving all the time, there are new methods of surgery and new materials, such as implants as well as innovations, such as 3D printing. Implants used in joint replacements now last longer than ever before and recovery

---

[16] Rheumatoid Arthritis and Surgery (2025) nras/resource/surgery

times have improved as more is understood about the best aftercare advice to give to patients".

In fact, there is evidence from a few studies showing that take up rates for surgery for RA have declined since peaking in the 1990s. Indeed, my consultant surgeon who performed my elbow replacement in 2024 said to me that he did not see many cases nowadays except for people like me with long standing RA that had started a long time ago.

My right elbow replacement went very well and was totally successful in reducing the pain from the elbow, which was caused by ulnar nerve entrapment. The elbow now has very good flexion and improved straightening and best of all no pain. I did have to wait ages for this operation though, as I was referred to two different hospitals where the orthopaedic consultants did not have the experience to perform an elbow replacement as there is less demand for them now. The third hospital had good expertise so in the end it was a great success.

It is good to know that most people with RA will not need this operation nowadays, but some people with RA might need hand surgery as RA most often starts in the hands and wrists. Hand surgery comes in many forms. Some people may need a synovectomy, the removal of inflamed tissue, which in turn reduces inflammation, pain and swelling. Other people may need operations like tendon repairs, or they may need joints, such as the finger joints, aligned. You could also have joints fused to reduce pain and joint replacements of the knuckles [MCP joints] are available if needed.

The damage to my hands was well underway before I was even diagnosed and my wrists fused themselves in my twenties and thirties. I did have a tendon transfer when a tendon snapped in my right thumb, but it wasn't very successful, my middle thumb joint has been fixed since then.

The MCP joint replacements came later - as did the alignment and correcting of deformities - so I have not had any of these done and I cannot remember them being offered to me before the 1990s when I felt it was too late.

Knee operations have been carried out successfully since the eighties though. It is a complicated joint, but the replacements are now lighter, and less bone is removed, so these replacements last well and are very successful. As noted before my own was done just before the covid lockdown, so I was very lucky indeed and after the initial swelling subsided it has been brilliant.

'I have not had foot surgery, but my ankles are fused as well as a couple of toes. I have kept walking by wearing supportive trainers with cushioned insoles but if I did need surgery on my feet or ankles then it would be much easier and more successful now in the 2020s than it was in the 70s and 80s.

NRAS [17] says on their website that surgery has a lot to offer the rheumatoid patient with foot and ankle problems and " in the last 25 years, there has been an explosion of interest in foot and ankle surgery, and there are now many orthopaedic surgeons in the UK who specialise in foot and ankle surgery. Newer techniques are therefore more widespread and

---

[17] Rheumatoid Arthritis and Surgery (2025) nras/resource/surgery

practised by a greater number of foot and ankle surgeons, providing more availability with a wider range of treatment options for the rheumatoid patient."

In summary it seems that surgery offers some good results but thankfully nowadays it is less needed, certainly in younger people. A study listed in the National Library of Medicine [18]showed that the rates of joint surgery in RA peaked in the 1990s and have since declined suggesting that long-term outcomes of RA are improving. This study tells us that rates of ankle and wrist surgery were markedly lower in the mid-2000s compared to the mid-1980s and rates of total knee arthroplasty and total hip arthroplasty also decreased substantially (19% and 40%, respectively) among patients aged 40–59 years.

So less people with RA need surgery nowadays but when they do need it then very good results are possible. So, the future is definitely a lot brighter for anyone diagnosed with RA now. Improved medications, better and safer surgery are the most important changes but there have been other improvements in the wider society too.

One of these changes is the availability of information, advice and support for newly diagnosed people with RA in comparison with the situation that I found myself in during the 70s and 80s. The internet has been developed during my life with RA and there are many more ways of finding out about RA,

[18] Louie G H, Ward M M, Changes in the rates of Joint Surgery among patients with Rheumatoid Arthritis in California, 1983-2007 https://www.ncbi.nlm.nih.gov/pmc/articles/PMC2859109/

the treatments available and the best ways to manage your condition.

Although there are many internet resources, I feel that NRAS is the very best online resource for people with RA as I discussed in Chapters 3 and 5. The information and the self-management modules they have produced are excellent as are the resources for those who are newly diagnosed. There is plenty of information on exercise as well, with a general module emphasising the importance of exercise and activity alongside six modules highlighting specific forms of exercise. These include Strengthening and Resistance, Tai Chi and Movement to Music.

Sometimes with RA, especially when it's invisible, it's hard for other people to understand the difficulties that you have, people can be very intolerant or impatient when they can't see your pain or frustration. NRAS has a helpline with volunteers who listen and understand, there are local groups and internet groups and a self-help health forum as well as lots of interesting articles on various subjects like gardening, flying, being a parent etc.

There are also reader stories which are very interesting and inspiring. You can be involved as little or as much as you wish but there is usually a need for volunteers to join in with surveys or research and many other roles. There is also an annual RA Awareness week which focuses on different areas of misconceptions.

Often, people think that RA is like osteo-arthritis, and it happens to old people. They just don't understand that it can affect the whole body and its' systems and it's most often young and middle-aged people who are diagnosed as well as some older people.

There is a wealth of information out there for those diagnosed with RA these days meaning that you can easily research medication, complementary therapies, diet and food information or the accessibility of places you want to visit. You can readily listen to inspiring and practical health blogs and podcasts.

Something else that has also made life easier for people with RA is the option of online shopping. It has been a godsend to me for the last twenty years since my accident in 2004. I decided to continue with it once I was recovered because it has been virtually impossible for me to go shopping for many years. I can't reach things, or grasp them if they are too wide, I can't stand in queues or lift heavy bags. The option to shop online keeps me independent and I really don't miss food shopping very much at all.

In the wider society there has been many legal changes that have helped people with disabilities. Some of this legislation is very helpful to people with RA who sometimes struggle with everyday activities. The following paragraphs cover some of the legal changes that have happened since 1974, when my RA started.

Personal Independence Payments [PIP] previously DLA, started in 1992.and this is a non means tested payment that is given to help with funding any extra needs that you may have when you have a long-term condition or disability. For instance, it could allow you to lower your working hours, pay for equipment that you need or fund a car or mobility scooter or perhaps you might need it to pay for some help in the home. Having a long-term condition does reduce your income if you are unable to work full time due to fatigue or pain, and so, with shorter hours and according to your financial situation, you may be able to claim some universal credit as well as PIP. In actual fact at the time of writing the government is looking for ways to reduce its welfare bill so hopefully there may be more support available to help people back to work if they have had to stop working when they were newly diagnosed but are ready to work now symptoms are well controlled. Also, there are now more jobs allowing home working since covid, so this option may also help you to return to work too. Of course, employment, aside from the income, provides social contacts, self-respect and the satisfaction of achievement, new learning and in some roles more physical activity. It also builds a structure to the day that many people find useful.

Another change in the law that was, and is, very helpful for people with RA was the Disability Discrimination Act in 1995 which made it illegal to discriminate against disabled people in employment or in the provision of good and services. As mentioned in an earlier chapter this particular piece of legislation enabled me to keep my job.

A person is defined as disabled when they have a physical or mental health condition or illness that has lasted or is expected to last 12 months or more, which reduces their ability to carry out day-to-day activities. This definition definitely includes people with RA, and it has meant that continuing employment is now more possible once reasonable adjustments are arranged by employers.

Also, the Discrimination Act has meant that service providers like shops, restaurants, cinemas and providers of public transport also have to make provision for people with disabilities. Before this act it was very difficult for some people to go out of their home without a great deal of planning and sometimes it was impossible depending on the disability. These days people with RA often don't see themselves as having a disability or being disabled and I certainly didn't until I was in my late forties. However, there can be times when people with RA do need to use a wheelchair or occasions when walking is reduced or slow and painful. At these times it's very helpful to have accommodations like level access, close parking, flexibility and reasonable adjustments at work as well as patience from the people around you!

In 1996 the Community Care [Direct payments] Act was passed. These payments are helpful if you are struggling with everyday tasks like eating, drinking, preparing food, dressing or showering. They can also be helpful or needing a P.A. to help with activities like attending exercise classes or shopping. The payments may help to fund someone to support you with gardening or essential cleaning in your house.

If your savings are under the social care threshold you can be assessed to receive direct payments to help fund essential needs, instead of or as well as having a care worker commissioned by Social Care [The rules around this vary according to how much budget the local council has for social care at the time and so what you are allowed to request varies according to what is seen as essential!] In the past when I was working as an OT, I allocated money for petrol for a car for essential journeys and activities, a P.A to accompany a client to swimming or exercise classes, payments for garden help or meal preparation as well as care workers for personal care assistance.

Something else that has changed is disability rights. Since 2000 there have been at least three important milestones which give people with disabilities, including people with long term or invisible conditions the right to be treated equally. These three laws are all helpful to people with RA as they are helping to break down barriers that people with disabilities sometimes face. Nowadays many of the physical barriers have been removed but there is still a way to go before people with disabilities are seen for who they are and not defined by their illness or disability in particular, people with disabilities should be seen as people first and foremost, and not as someone with a disability.

Social and cultural attitudes and assumptions about people with impairments perpetuate prejudice, discrimination and exclusion in society. For instance [19] "assumptions that people with certain impairments can't work, can't be independent, can't have sex, shouldn't have children, need protecting, are "child-like", are " dangerous", should not be seen because they are upsetting, or are scroungers." More people with disabilities in the community or being portrayed positively in all types of media like TV, films, YouTube etc would really help to remove

---

[19] Attitudinal Barriers,(2025) https://www.inclusionlondon.org.uk/about-us/disability-in-london/social-model/the-social-model-of-disability

these attitudinal barriers that need to be broken down.

Since the introduction of the Disability Discrimination Act [DDA] in 1995 many things have improved in the UK, but more improvement is still needed. Society is going in the right direction, but the process takes time, we should not be satisfied until every person is treated with the respect they deserve. In relation to RA the future is so much brighter now for anyone who has recently had a diagnosis. There is a much better choice of medications, vastly improved surgery, more diagnostic scans and tests as well as much more availability of information, guidance and support.

Chapter 8: Achieving a Positive Outlook

I have written this second book to encourage people with R.A. to take more control of their life, by finding ways of solving their problems, learning about their condition and generally helping themselves to achieve a more positive outlook.

I also wanted to demonstrate how much more positive the future is if you have RA diagnosed nowadays. Even so it may still feel like a shock when you first receive the news that you have a long-term condition with no cure. In order to become more positive, it is necessary to have some understanding of the psychological effects of chronic conditions.

The psychological aspects are important because they can prevent us from accepting our situation, making changes and taking control of our lives. People are very different and deal with the diagnosis in a variety of ways but nevertheless some generalisations can still be made. I would like to end this book with the same chapter that ended my first book 20 years ago as it is still as relevant today.

Dealing with your diagnosis

I started thinking about how I had felt all those years ago and then I began to realise that what I had experienced when I found out that I had RA were actually the stages of grief. During my

O.T. training we learnt about these stages of grief in connection with bereavement but equally they also apply to other losses that we may experience in our lives when we have a chronic deteriorating condition. Having R.A. definitely feels like a loss because you feel that you will lose your future as an active, fit, healthy person. It is not what you had planned for your life. As well as the loss of health and energy you begin to think of other losses.

For instance, you may worry that if you cannot work you will lose money and all the things that it can buy as well as losing your self-esteem and confidence. You may feel that RA will make you a less attractive person if you end up with deformities or swollen joints. You might also worry about losing friends if you do not feel well enough to go out and socialise. Going through the stages of grief is therefore a very normal thing to do considering the uncertain future. We need to go through these stages to be able to move on and reach the last stage of acceptance. It is then possible to make changes and develop new skills and interests and generally get on with life.

How we deal with loss

You may feel a sense of shock and disbelief, and this will happen when you first learn that you have RA. Alternatively it could be a relief if you were expecting worse news or had no diagnosis previously. Sometimes it is reassuring to realise that there is a reason for the way that you feel. I felt upset in the first few weeks and months and wanted to keep talking about it and this is the way I expressed my feelings. Some of you may act in a different way by crying or by feeling that you do not really have

RA and it must all be a mistake.

Why me?

The next reaction is often "why me" why should I have to deal with this disabling condition, what have I done to deserve this? This is a very normal and understandable reaction; it is part of the second stage of grief. It is very reasonable to feel a certain amount of self-pity if you have a chronic condition with no cure, because you may feel that there are many things that you will now never be able to achieve in your life. It will also feel unfair to have to put up with pain and very unfair to have RA at all and all this could make you feel angry.

Anger

There are many other reasons for feeling angry too. You may be angry because you cannot keep a job or obtain one. You may be angry and upset because you are not able to do all the things that you want to. Some people may feel annoyed that their partners or family are not helping them enough or that their work colleagues do not understand. Anger is also part of the second stage of grief and resentment of others is also a part of this.

Depression

In some cases, suppressed anger can lead to depression. Studies have found that the prevalence of clinical depression in patients with RA is higher than that of the general population.

Anyone with depression will be unable to motivate him or herself to get on with life or to make changes. It is therefore important to seek help early on if you find yourself becoming very negative about everything. Discussing problems and trying to find some solutions to at least some of them will help to prevent a deterioration of mental health.

Denial

Another common problem, which can reduce the effectiveness of treatment, is denial of reality or focusing only on obtaining a cure. Denial is a way of protecting yourself from unpleasant truths and future worries and it is also a part of the second stage of grief. It is true that too much information too soon can promote anxiety and fear, but denying to yourself that you have the condition can prevent you from getting on with life and making the necessary changes now. Although it is necessary to have some hope of improvement, awaiting a miracle cure or waiting for health professionals to produce a magical solution is counterproductive. In any case there is no answer to the 'why me' question and there is at present no complete cure. RA cannot be attributed to diet or lifestyle or anything that you could have brought on yourself. It is important to remember that RA. is not a life-threatening disease and symptoms can be improved a lot. A very good quality of life is still possible with a few adjustments.

Becoming an expert patient

Discuss any problems that you have whether they are

connected to work, daily living tasks, social life, hobbies, and family or sex life. Ask about medication or gain more information on the condition. Talk to a health professional or a friend or family member. Look up information in books, on web sites or in leaflets or just keep asking questions. If you have problems at work think about the changes you would like to make and discuss them with a manager or access to work or both. Be proactive and do not give up. Having information will help you makes decisions and achieve goals. Seeking information and trying to make sense of the situation is the third stage of grief and it will hopefully lead onto the last stage of acceptance.

The stages of grief do not follow an exact pattern. Some stages overlap with others, sometimes we go back a stage, we do not necessarily experience all of them. Some people experience a stage of depression after the third stage because they cannot make sense of what is happening, they cannot see any future at this time. Eventually most of us will move on to acceptance and begin a new future.

The benefits of active coping

Seeking information is an active coping mechanism and many studies have shown that people who have active coping mechanisms feel less helpless, tend to exhibit fewer symptoms and generally have a greater sense of well-being. An investigation by Parker et al [20] in 1988 studied 84 patients with

---

[20] Parker, J *et al* (1988) *Journal of Rheumatology*, Sept; 15(9): 1376-83

RA. The investigation looked at functional status i.e. your ability to manage activities, coping style, the activity of the disease and pain. Parker found out that patients who coped by restructuring life goals had better functional status and psychological adjustment than patients who hoped for unrealistic solutions or engaged in blaming themselves for the illness. A study by Bendtsen and Hornquist [21] in Sweden examined clinical well-being and coping on 222 patients with R.A. Those who had accepted the illness showed less guilt and tension and more endurance, and those who had decided on an active life showed a more positive belief in the future- which of course is important for good health and well-being.

Positive thinking

Another active coping mechanism is cognitive restructuring. This is the idea of changing your thinking patterns so that you interpret events and outcomes in a more positive way rather than tending to focus on the negative. If you are thinking negatively about a situation, try and look at the situation in another way. Many situations and events can be viewed in a more positive light. You must see the half-filled glass as half full and not as half empty! Do not expect yourself to be one of the few people with RA who ends up in a wheelchair with many disabilities and totally dependent. This is called catastrophising and people who catastrophise believe in the worst possible

[21] Bentsen, P and Hornquist, JO (1994) *Scandinavian Journal of Social Medicine*, June;22(2):87-106

outcome for their future and become negative in their thoughts. It is important that patients with RA do not catastrophise. A study by Keefe et al [22] showed that patients who catastrophised tended to have poorer outcomes in terms of pain, physical disability and depression.

Helpful support

A lot of studies have researched the importance of social support from close friends or family. Social support is about relationships with others and how these can improve your health and well-being. This type of support can be effective in helping to prevent depression.

It is not necessary to have a large number of friends, but it is necessary to have the type of support that you need. If people are over supportive, they can take over all your roles and do everything for you and this is not helpful. It is actually detrimental because you are likely to become physically weaker as well as gradually losing your confidence and self-esteem. You will eventually stop being involved in your own life! The support that is beneficial is the type that can be called upon when it is needed and what you want will depend on your lifestyle and what you are able to manage.

Riemsma et al [23] in the Netherlands examined fatigue in people with RA in relation to the type of support that they received. They studied the levels of fatigue in relation to how

---

[22] Keefe, F *et al* (1989) *Pain*, 37: 51-6
[23] Riemsma, RP *et al* (1998) *British Journal of Rheumatology*, Oct; 37(10):1042-6

people managed their support networks, the activity of their disease and demographic [population] variables. The result was that patients who took control of their support networks and could call on them when they were required had less fatigue, whilst those with problematic support had more fatigue. [problematic support is support that does not suit your needs] This shows that support is only helpful when it is doing just that, helping you when it is needed. This allows you to get on with your life in your own way. Social support must not take over your life and reduce you to total dependency.

What support do you need?

The support that is needed may take the form of practical assistance or helping out with suggestions; or it could involve listening to your frustrations and just being there for you. Some people might prefer a therapist or counsellor when they feel the need to offload, rather than discussing issues with a partner or friend who is involved in the situation. It is really up to you to decide what suits you.

The support that you need will also depend on your physical abilities and the pain you experience. Severity of disease is not necessarily the most significant factor affecting your physical ability or the pain that is experienced. Other psychological factors play a part.

This has been shown to be the case in quite a few studies

including one by Hagglund et al [24] in 1989. Disease severity and coping strategies were examined to see if they predicted the degree of pain and physical impairments that would be experienced. The severity of disease demonstrated no significant relationship to the measure of outcome i.e. pain and physical abilities.

This shows that the way that you cope is just as important as the seriousness of the disease when it comes to predicting how much pain or loss of abilities will occur. The best way to manage is to readjust life goals and your work and activities. Always find a new way forward and look for the positive.

Being positive is beneficial for health

Being positive has been shown to be very beneficial for health. Martin Seligman [25] has studied optimism and pessimism extensively and he has observed that pessimists are more prone to depression and more likely to have poor health. Optimistic and pessimistic attitudes seem to be set early on in life and are the result of how we are made, how we are treated and what events happen in our formative years.

It is possible to try and become more optimistic by interpreting situations in a more positive way. Many events can be viewed in different ways, for instance, if you have failed an exam you can choose to believe that you failed because you

---

[24] Hagglund, KJ *et al* (1989) *Arthritis and Rheumatism*, July; 32(7) ;851-8

[25] Seligman, M (11998) Learned optimism, in Manning, M, *The Healing Journey*. Piatkus

were unlucky, all the wrong questions came up; or that the paper was much harder than usual. You could also take the view that your failure was because you did not do enough work or that you are not really clever enough to be doing this exam and there is no use trying again. These are all possible interpretations, and some are more pessimistic than others. Optimists will move on and find a new way forward or a reason to be positive. They will try not to feel helpless or hopeless. The way to be an optimist is to make realistic goals that you can achieve and to look at all the interpretations for a situation and use the positive ones. Achat et al [26] studied optimism and depression as predictors of physical and mental health functioning. They found out that optimism is associated with higher levels of general health perceptions, vitality and mental health and lower levels of pain.

Coming to terms with R.A.... my own experience

Some people are happy to depend on others, but most people like to be as independent as possible. It is particularly difficult to request help when you are young. I found that when I went shopping, I often couldn't reach items, it was very difficult for me to pack bags quickly enough at the till. It was difficult for me to ask for help because no-one could really see that I had a disability; you cannot see weakness and pain.

Later on, as my hands became more deformed the opposite happened. People either tried to do too much or

---

[26] Achat, H *et al* (2000) *Annals of Behavioural Medicine*, Spring; 22(2):127-30

looked embarrassed or stared at my hands. I do not really have a problem with this now as I just ask for help if I need it and say "no thanks, it's OK" if I don't need it.

Of course, it is easy for me to be able to say this now because I have had the condition for over 50 years, and it takes time to adjust to having RA or any debilitating chronic condition. I have gone through many stages in my life. At first, I ignored the intense pain and carried on regardless. Then my doctor gave me anti-inflammatory drugs but because he did not let me know that I had a chronic condition I continued to try and ignore the pain.

Nearly ten years later I decided that I wanted answers, and I asked for them. On receiving the diagnosis, I continually needed to talk about it. I was quite angry at the way I was told. Everything seemed to be so very negative, things would get worse, I would lose the rest of my wrist movement etc.

Over the next few months I searched for information, as much as I could cope with. I attended the O.T department. I was given the time to ask questions about medication or talk about practical problems. I learnt exercises to maintain as much strength and range of movements as I could. I learnt about posture and joint protection and many other things that I have written about in this book. Mostly I became aware that it is possible to have a chronic disease but also be in good health.

I have concluded my book with this section about psychology because I feel that it is definitely possible to have good health and well-being whilst having a chronic illness. In order to achieve the best outcome, it is important to help yourself and take responsibility for your health.

The medical profession can offer some assistance but there are many decisions for you to take. There are also many ways to help yourself.

- Firstly, you need to be informed about your condition. You then need to keep yourself as physically fit as possible so that your joints and muscles remain as strong as possible.
- Secondly, find work and leisure occupations that you enjoy and are able to manage.
- Thirdly look after your social contacts; friends and family are important.
- Lastly have fun and be optimistic.

The cards you have been given may not be the best but there are undoubtedly worst hands and it's the way you play your hand that counts.

Appendix

Good Posture

As well as doing exercise it is important to ensure that you have good posture. This is particularly important for anyone with RA because the pain or discomfort that occurs tends to make us avoid certain positions and movements. This means that if, for instance, your right foot hurts then you will put more weight on the left one, or if your neck hurts you may hold your head in a tilted position without realising it. In either case the body is not working in its natural way, and the spine will be compensating to keep the body in balance. This can cause back problems and/or damage to the joint that is working harder i.e. the left foot or the neck in the instances mentioned above.

Avoidance of any particular movement for prolonged periods means that the ligaments and tendons in the affected area will shorten because they are not being used fully. This means, for instance, if you were to remain sitting in a wheelchair for months and you never straightened your legs out, then the tendons would gradually shorten, the knees would become contracted and then it would become impossible to stand. This is why it is vital to put all joints through their normal range of movements [or as much as you can manage] regularly and to try as far as possible to ensure correct posture at all times. A physiotherapist or occupational therapist will be able to give advice on this. Alternatively, it may be worthwhile paying privately for a practitioner who can advise you on the Alexander technique, particularly if bad habits have been already formed for a long time.

The Alexander technique teaches you to be aware of your body and to think about the way that you are carrying out physical actions. The practitioner will guide you and make you aware of incorrect postures and in this way, you will improve the body's alignment. This will then prevent bad posture, muscle tension and pain.

Guidelines for good posture

Standing

Always ensure that your head is not tilted to the left or to the right, forwards or backwards. Look in the mirror to make sure you are looking straight ahead. If your head is carried correctly then it is more likely that weight will be spread through your body correctly. If your weight is not distributed properly then this will place a strain on your joints. Stand so that your weight is placed equally through both feet. The ankles, knees, hips and shoulders should be in line when standing. [If possible do not stand for too long].

Wear supportive shoes that give arch support and support to the inside of the foot. Push off from the heels and roll onto the toes. Try and keep a spring in the step if at all possible. Do not walk with the head down. Ensure the head is in a balanced position as in standing.

Sitting

Sit on a chair of the correct seat height so that your back is supported, and your feet are flat on the floor. An armrest and headrest are useful. You should sit up straight and not slump down however you should relax the shoulders. It is important to choose furniture that is supportive, firm and comfortable. If you have short legs, you may find that many chairs have too greater distance from the back to the front of the seat and it is therefore difficult to support your back and reach the floor without curving your back. Shop around and find one that is suitable for you, it will be well worth the time spent.

Lying down.

Have a mattress that is firm but also feels soft. Use a pillow that just cushions the curve at the neck, it should not be too high, and you should not use two unless you have some sort of breathing problems. Ensure that the bed is of an appropriate height to get in and out of easily. This will prevent strain on the knees and hips when you get out.

Working at a worktop or desk.

The desk should be of an appropriate height so that you do not have to lean forward. Your arm should be supported when writing. A speaker on your phone or mobile is essential if you have to do a lot of phone work or use headphones.

Kitchen work tops should be of an appropriate height. You need the surface lower for hard work e.g. mixing a cake but higher for chopping and lighter work.

Whatever you are doing remember to change positions frequently. You should not sit at a keyboard for more than 20-30 minutes. Stand up and walk across the room or office, stretch your fingers, roll your shoulders. This will prevent you from getting stiff and will allow you to move more easily.

If you have unsuitable furniture and equipment at your workplace you could give "Access to Work" a try. This is a scheme that can be used to fund adaptations to your workplace if you have a disability. [See chapter 4]

Joint Protection

Joint protection is an alternative method of carrying out everyday tasks, which will reduce the strain on your joints and therefore reduce pain. Using these techniques will also help to minimise joint deformities. Joint protection is sometimes taught as a group session at an Occupational Therapy department, or it could be taught individually. It involves both formal teaching and practical applications. People often enjoy being in a group as they can then encourage each other and swap ideas. It may be the case that this is the first opportunity that people with RA have had to talk to others with RA.

In order to achieve the optimum results, it is necessary to incorporate the new ideas on a daily basis. This will take quite a lot of thought initially but later on, if practised regularly, it will become automatic. If joint protection is incorporated into the daily routine, then significant benefits should result.

There are three main principles involved in joint protection, and they are listed below.

1 Conserving your energy
2 Avoiding static positions
3 Discouraging deformities

1 Conserving your energy

Having RA means that you are likely to have less energy than the average person when the RA is active. It also means that your joints are much more vulnerable to damage than other people's joints are. You therefore need to be organised and only do things that are absolutely necessary or things that are important to you. This is particularly necessary if you have a flare up and feel very tired. How much can be left undone depends on the situation you are in.

It is better to try and organise your life so that on an average day it is possible to fit in everything you want to do with time to spare. This means not taking on too much and being realistic in what you decide to achieve. In fact, this should apply to everyone not just people with RA. Try and spread the workload evenly over the week or month so that there is an even balance of more physical activities and more restful ones. For example, it is not a good idea to clean all the windows on the same day, but it is better to do one per day or one a week. Equally it is not a good choice to sit at a computer all day. Even if you are looking after young children it is possible to vary the activities carried out in any one day and incidentally this is much better for the children too. You can do some physical activities but sit down and enjoy a game or read a book or watch some TV in between the demanding tasks.

Think about the type of work you do because it may be possible to alter the planning of the day or build in rests. It might even be a good idea to change the type of work altogether if it is continually putting strain on the same joints or making you very tired. Start by analysing your working day and deciding what can be eliminated, if anything and find a beneficial pattern of activity and rest for what remains. Ensure that you do some physical tasks because it is important to exercise to keep muscles strong. It is the balance of activity and rest that is essential. Prioritise and schedule the most important issues first. Sometimes we put too higher expectations and standards on ourselves. Some tasks can be left undone without it really mattering too much; after all, health is the most important issue.

It is also important to think about the way you do tasks and the postures that you adopt for them because you could be placing more strain on your joints or taking more effort than you need to be. Is there an easier way to carry out this activity? Could it be done less often? Alternatively, could someone else be doing it?

I practise energy conservation and the way that I did this when I was working was by spreading my work hours over five days and working about five hours daily. I could do this because luckily, I did not have to work fulltime. After work and at weekends I tended to do a mixture of physical activities like housework, cooking, walking the dog, swimming, shopping, light gardening and some restful ones like reading, singing, listening to music, telephoning, watching T.V, socialising and when the children were younger doing various activities with them. I never did more than two hours of anything, I took coffee breaks frequently! Occasionally I went out for a day and did more walking than usual and often I ended up paying the price later in the day or the next day. It is still worth it on the odd occasion if you really want to do something special.

2 Avoiding static positions.

A static position is one that involves using the same set of muscles continually rather than alternating the groups of muscles used. For instance, if you sit and hold up a newspaper this places the shoulder muscles in a static position, however, swinging your arms while you are walking is an action that involves continually changing the muscle groups. It places more strain on a joint to continually use it in the same way and it also uses more energy to maintain a static position.

Anyone with RA needs to continually change positions to avoid repeated strain on particular joints. This means alternating between standing, sitting, walking and lying down. It also means that if you are working using your finger joints then your next action should preferably involve the use of different joints, or the same joints used in a different way.

For instance, if you are mixing a cake then this involves a beating motion with the hands and most of the strain is on the elbows and shoulders and wrists so the next task should use the hands in a different way. You could change to typing because this is using the fingers, wrists and shoulders in a different way, but it would be even better to walk the dog or sit down and read because this would be a complete change of activity involving different joints. Gentle movements of the joints seem to be best because they stop the joints stiffening but do not strain them. I find that small amounts of light washing up are actually very beneficial. The warm water and gentle movements make the joints feel more comfortable.

Carrying out activities around the house is more beneficial than a very long walk providing they are not too strenuous. This is because the movement loosens off the stiffness but does not cause pain. If you need to sit down for a long time, then get up and stretch your legs every 20 minutes or so. It is always a good idea to change positions every 20-30 minutes if you are able to.

3 Discouraging deformities

In RA the first joints to be affected are usually the fingers, wrists and toes. The overproduction of fluid results in the ligaments becoming loose and then these joints are likely to move in an abnormal way. Inflammation sometimes also causes the tendons to weaken. Joint damage means that some movements are restricted. This restriction combined with the loose ligaments, weak tendons and the swelling of the joints means that affected joints are then used in abnormal ways to compensate. For instance, if the wrist movement is reduced then finger joints are more likely to take up abnormal positions to counteract this e.g. the finger joints drift and the fingers become angled towards the little finger. This is called ulnar drift. Care is needed so that the fingers are not encouraged to take up these positions. Putting pressure on joints also makes deformity more likely. Joint protection procedures will not stop these things happening, but they will slow down the process. Using the joints in as normal way as possible also means that if joints do fuse because of cartilage damage then they will fuse in a normal working position and therefore it will still be possible to carry out many actions.

Avoid actions that encourage deformity.

Opening jars, screwing lids, turning taps and holding plates can encourage deformities in the hands. You should hold a dinner plate either with two hands or by using the palm of the hand. It is also better to use the palms of the hand when opening jars or bottles. If you have to perform a turning or twisting movement using the fingers always ensure that the fingers are being encouraged to move towards the thumb and not towards the little finger. This means learning to use both hands is very useful. For example, you should turn on a tap with your right hand and turn it off with your left one. You could use a special jar opener to allow the jar to be opened more easily. Use a wall tin opener for tins if they do not have a ring pull opener. Never pull open ring pull cans with one finger, use a knife to lever it open or use a special ring pull opener. Finger joints can also be placed into positions of deformity by pushing up on the knuckles or leaning the chin onto the hands. Both these positions should be avoided. Reading a book by holding it up in one hand can put strain on the finger joints. It is better to rest the book on the table or use a bookrest or draw up the knees and rest it on them.

Avoid tight grips

It places more pressure on the joints to pick up small items than larger ones therefore handles on utensils should be larger to reduce the strain. It is therefore better to use mugs with thick handles rather than elegant china teacups with dainty handles. Spreading your fingers around the mug is a much better position for the finger joints but always wait until the drink has cooled or use an insulated mug. Use kitchen tools and cutlery with chunkier handles rather than slim ones. If you are using a knife ensure that it is sharp, this reduces the power needed to cut. There are special right-angled knives that can also be used as they reduce the power needed. It is useful to use a pen that is thicker or a pen grip particularly if you intend to write for long periods of time although less writing is done these days.

Use a larger joint or several joints rather than small joints

If you are carrying objects like saucepans and plates then use two hands, using one hand will place that hand in a position of deformity. You can buy dishes, casseroles and saucepans with two handles on. It is useful to use a tray to carry items but make sure that it has suitable handles at each side. Use a baking tray to put casseroles or cakes on.

It is never a good idea to carry heavy loads and certainly not on one or two fingers. Shopping bags should be carried over the arm or over the shoulder and they should not be too heavy. Alternatively, they can be carried close to the body in a bag or rucksack. It is always better to spread loads over more joints or use larger joints. Use a car or home delivery wherever possible or otherwise a trolley rather than carry weights like shopping bags for long distances.

Choose suitable equipment.

Using lightweight equipment will reduce the strain on joints. There are lighter options for most equipment whether it is for kitchen use or for DIY or for housework. If you are buying new equipment or being given a present choose with the weight in mind rather than just going for looks. Choose fittings that can easily be operated like levers rather than knobs e.g. choose lever taps in place of crystal or traditional four prong taps.

Occupational therapists will give all this information to their patients if they are referred for therapy. I was not referred until I already had many deformities and therefore, I did not know about joint protection until I had had RA for at least ten years. I therefore did all the wrong things for a very long time. It is likely that I would have suffered a lot less pain if I had practised joint protection earlier on.

In my life I have had to learnt to negotiate in order that I can experience less pain and stiffness although this does not mean that I have been prepared to give up everything that I enjoy. There have been many times when I have chosen to ignore joint protection and conservation of energy because I had wanted to achieve a personal goal however I only ignore it for an extremely good reason. At 39 I had never achieved my ambition of going ski-ing and for a week. I put my principles on hold and punished my joints and also risked a few broken bones. I did some exercise before I went and luckily my bones survived intact. It was well worth the risk to achieve an ambition. I really enjoyed the opportunity to ski.

Generally, though, since being aware of joint protection, I am a lot more careful, I mostly follow the guidelines and have also found my own ways to make my life easier and to protect my joints. In the kitchen my cooker is near to the sink, I can slide saucepans along. I can then tip them from the edge of the sink into a colander without the need to lift them. I took a lot of care whenever I bought a cooker ensuring that I could use the controls. The knobs an optimum size and easy to turn and the oven self- cleaning inside and now I have a touch sensitive hob and oven. These priorities came before being fashionable or having the colour or model that I preferred. Within the price range it usually means that I effectively have very little choice!

All the taps in my house are very easy to use and if any equipment is due to be replaced, I always choose very light items. Most of my pots and pans have two handles or are very light and I am still able to cook meals for two, although for some I need help. We have a light vacuum cleaner.

On the whole once you have learnt the principles of joint protection you will find ways of incorporating them into your own lifestyle. I have my own way of peeling potatoes. I put them onto the surface, holding them still with one hand and then I use a sharp knife to peel downwards. I do not hold the potatoes in my hand because it is uncomfortable and encourages deformity. I have drawers that can slide open easily and I use appropriate heights to prepare food. I also have a small jug kettle or otherwise use both hands when I lift a larger kettle. I use a plastic jug to fill the kettle. Sometimes specialised equipment is necessary to assist with reducing deformities and the reduction of strain on the joints and I have a few items that I regularly use. Openers for tins and jars, right angled knives, a travel kettle, thicker handles on cutlery. In the next section there are some ideas to help with everyday activities if you have a period of pain, stiffness or swelling of you have joint damage or are recovering from an operation.

Tips and Ideas for Easier Living

In the last update of my original book, I decided to add in a new section. The idea arose because I realised that in my own home or out in my own car, I am almost totally independent but when I am at other houses or in a hotel or away anywhere new, I feel very disabled. It is the environment that makes me feel that way and it's not nice. I have added it in again and ensured that it's up to date.

There are many things that are or have been difficult or impossible for me. Here are some of my immediate thoughts.

- Hanging my coat on a hook and getting it off afterwards
- Opening cupboards and also being able to reach right in and take out items that I need
- Opening drawers or turning on taps
- Reaching plug sockets to switch on electric equipment
- Reaching hangers in wardrobes
- Making meals or even drinks
- Opening containers or taking things out of containers
- Going up or down the stairs or going up or down steep slopes and ramps
- Getting off a very low chair. I have to remember not to sit in it in the first place!
- Having a shower or bath
- Cutting up meat

- Using metal cutlery
- Locking the toilet door in case I cannot get out again!

I have gathered together some tips and ideas that may be helpful to others. Some I have used as a therapist, others I use myself and quite a few have come from the members of NRAS. All these suggestions have been tested out either by myself or by other people with RA.

Personal Care

Shampoo blocks/ bars are often easier to use than bottles of shampoo. See for instance Lush or Body shop or Holland & Barrett Faith in nature.

If you have difficulties when reaching **to wash under your arms**, use a long handled washing up mop and place a flannel over it.

Use a **spong**e to wash rather than a flannel as it's easier to squeeze it out.

Using a **bath lift, bath board or bath seat** helps you to use the bath if you are unable to get out.

A **long-handled sponge or loofah** is useful for reaching all over your body.

A **raised toilet seat** is the answer for those days when it's really painful to get up and down from the toilet. It is removable.

Use bubble bath. Then there's no need to clean the bath

separately after use, just spray it.

Buy **empty soap dispensers** and fill them with shampoo or conditioner if you have problems squeezing bottles.

Alternatively leave shower gel and shampoo bottles upside down so that the liquid comes out more easily.

Drying yourself after a bath

Try using a **towelling tea towel**, which is light, absorbent and will easily bend into creases and under arms.

Use **cotton buds** to dry between the toes or use a hair dryer or a long-handled toe towel may help.

Use a **towelling dressing gown** after a bath or shower to ensure you are dry.

Get someone to stitch the two short sides of two bath towels together, leaving a hole for your head. This is useful when shoulders movement is limited.

Applying lotion: It can be very difficult to apply lotions to the body if you have damage to the hip joints or the wrists. Instead of buying a purpose made lotion applicator try a long-handled wooden spoon (smooth with no splintery bits) to do the job. Just squeeze the lotion onto the back of spoon and apply.

Brushing out hair If you have RA and you have restricted joint movement and poor grip it can be a painful experience to brush and comb out you own hair or your children's hair. **The Tangle**

Teezer is very easy to grip, and it glides through tangled hair effortlessly. It also gives you a relaxing head massage at the same time!

Widening the toothbrush handle. Put rubber bands round your toothbrush handle so it doesn't slip through your fingers if they feel stiff in the morning

Use light **plastic disposable razors** if shavers are too hard to lift and hold.

Use a **makeup sponge** it's easier on the skin too.

Squeeze toothpaste out by pressing down on the tube with your lower arm.

Clothing

Wear **stretchy fabrics** they are easier to take off.

Thermal fingerless gloves are useful for inside and outside the house if it's difficult to wear gloves with fingers. It also helps to protect the finger joints from knocks.

A piece of **ribbon or cord tied to a zip fastener** can make it easier to grip and to pull up and down.

Use a **dressing stick** to lift clothing off the shoulders or to pull clothing up. It's also useful to reach things.

Buy your clothes without **small fiddly buttons.**

Replace awkward buttons with Velcro (if you have to dress young children you may want to do this for some of their clothes as well).

Leggings are easier to put on than tights and are great with long skirts and boots.

Wearing a cape or a woollen wrap instead of a coat. It is so much easier to take off.

Lacing up shoes

You can buy **elastic laces** if it's difficult and fiddly to do up laces on your footwear.

You can also buy **coiled shoelaces.**

Cooking and Eating

Battery operated jar openers and can openers. One touch (the first widely available battery-operated tin opener) seems to be a favourite.

A **ring pull** is a useful gadget that lifts the rings up on cans and gets them open.

Try using **nut crackers** (the type with inside serrations) to unscrew small bottle tops.

Using a Cheese Grater To save the wrist strain that you get with vertical tower graters use a cheese grater that fits over a plastic bowl with a non-slip rubber ring underneath. The bowl also comes with a lid so you can store your grated cheese, carrots, etc.

Wide grip cutlery is a must for weak fingers as there is much less pressure on the joints.

Perching stools are great for the kitchen when you need to keep getting up and down or use any seat really. If there's not much space use a metal frame folding dining chair.

The **freezer** is so handy to make up meals, then they are ready for difficult days.

Lifting dishes out of the oven is easier and better for the wrist and finger joints if the dish is placed on a baking tray so that it can be lifted in and out with two hands.

You can also remove heavy items from the oven by placing a trolley beside the oven and lifting the dish with both hands onto the trolley. Then do a second lift onto the work surface (a metal trolley is preferable due to the risk of burning or marking a wooden trolley).

Use a **light tray** to carry cups and plates with both hands rather than struggling to lift them in your hands or carry items using both hands.

Two handled saucepans, frying pans and casseroles make life easier and reduce damage and strain on the joints.

Right angled easy grip knives make chopping and slicing much easier.

If china is too heavy try lightweight **Melamine tableware.**

When **cutting dried fruit**, e.g. apricots use scissors, rather than a knife, to make the job much easier.

Buy a **potato peeler with a wide grip handle** or better still cook potatoes with the skins on.

Use a steak knife rather than an ordinary knife when cutting meat. Take one with you when you go to a restaurant for a meal otherwise someone else may have to chop up your food!

Always keep your chopping knives sharp. It is much easier to chop food.

A **food processor** is a brilliant invention it saves so much pain and strain!

Garlic Use garlic paste, garlic granules or a bottle of concentrated garlic like very lazy garlic and very lazy ginger; so much easier than chopping!

Using a steamer means that you don't need to lift pans of water and strain vegetables. If you don't have a steamer, you could use a cooking basket.

Boil in the bag or microwavable rice is much easier to prepare. No need to drain or ask anyone else to drain it.

Buy an **electric mixer** for any baking /whisking.

Baby Bottles If you have a baby and use bottles, release the air by pressing the teat down. This makes the bottle easier to open.

Making drinks

A small **travel kettle** is great for making drinks for 1-2 people, alternatively use a kettle tipper.

The **Breville 'Hot Cup'** is useful for making drinks by pressing a button rather than lifting a heavy kettle. It can be refilled with a plastic jug.

The **Dolce Gusto coffee machine** is also easy to use. Just drop in a sachet, place the cup under and press.

Fill a kettle by using a **lightweight plastic jug** and only use a minimal amount of water.

Always use a **mug with a wide handle** and not a cup.

Walking and Driving

If you wear **thin driving gloves**, contact with the steering wheel is improved so there is less need to grip so hard.

Place a silk scarf or plastic bag on the driver or passenger seat of your car and you will **swivel with ease** if it is difficult getting in or out of the car.

Insoles can be useful for people with RA as they often walk on their heels and end up with pain at the back of the foot. The Busy Feet insoles are half insoles that cushion the heel really well and have a gentle arch support.

An **umbrella can be used as a walking stick** on difficult days. Alternatively use a ski pole.

Getting **petrol for the car** can be very difficult. Ask a local garage with more than one member of staff to serve you with fuel or, if you can, buy an electric car and charge from your own charging point.

It's a good idea never to overload a bag, just keep to the minimum like a purse or wallet, keys, mobile and tissues! Wear a crossover bag.

Buy a car with an **adjustable driving seat** so that your posture is better when driving.

Before buying a new car be a real pain. Try the keys in the ignition, open the doors and the boot, try moving the seat forward and back and up and down, ensure you can use all the switches and levers and make sure you can manage the gears and handbrake.

An automatic car is much easier if you have RA. It's definitely worth the extra money.

A **shopping trolley** may be useful to save carrying otherwise do your **shopping on the internet** when you can.

Other practical everyday ideas

A **wash-up sponge or washing up brush** can be much easier to squeeze and wash up rather than using a cloth.

A dish washer may be easier still however the warm water is therapeutic!

When you are unable to reach and bend **an "easy reacher"** is useful for helping with dressing, reaching items in cupboards or on the floor, and the hook at the end is useful to pull down blinds.

When buying a **vacuum cleaner** buy a light model like a Bissell light vacuum cleaner or a lightweight Dyson.

Have a **cordless phone** or mobile phone with a speaker so that you don't need to hold it.

Use a headset or headphones with your mobile phone.

Plug pulls can be fitted onto existing plugs so that you can get them in and out of the sockets more easily.

Change plugs on existing equipment that you use frequently to **"handiplugs"** plugs with the handle built in.

A **steam ironing press** takes all the hard work out of ironing.

Use **felt tips or thick, chunky pencils** for writing as there is less pressure on the finger and thumb joints.

Use **wide grip pens** or a **pen grip** around a thinner pen.

Request **easy open medication bottles** as the childproof ones are impossible to open.

Dusting: Use a clean dish mop as a duster for working in awkward corners and behind furniture. It saves moving heavy items.

Wrist supports: These pads can be comfortable and supportive when typing and relieve pressure on the wrist or OTs can provide working splints.

To help reduce wrist ache, wear an **elasticised woollen sports wrist band** (sold in pairs).

Folding trolleys or plastic boxes on wheels can have many uses, such as carrying shopping from the car, or moving laundry in the house.

To **widen handles,** use plastic tubing that will fit over the handle snuggly. If it is slightly loose apply some silicone adhesive (available from craft shops] and allow 24 hrs to set.

For extra grip on rails in your bathroom, cover rails with cycle tape, available in many colours from Halfords etc.

When you are unable to grip, ensure your hands are dry and also use a piece of kitchen towel to help.

Ensure washers are changed on taps so they don't need to be turned off hard.

Change taps to **lever taps,** so easy to turn and available in all

DIY shops.

Change door handles from knobs to levers, much easier to open.

Key or knob turners can be a good idea for yale type locks.

The **Magnetic Wand** tools picks up any screws, nails, drawing pins or metal bits that fall into corners where you can't easily reach.

Ensure drawers run in and out easily

Use a **shopping bag with long handles** so that you can carry shopping over your shoulder or arm to save the finger joints.

If bending down to pick up the mail is painful or difficult, fit a **letter box cage/catcher** to the inside of your door, under the letterbox.

Use **chair or bed raisers** if you have to struggle to get up.

If you have trouble fastening bracelets and necklaces try some with **magnet clasps.**

An **electric 'under-blanket'** for your bed can be useful to soothe aching, stiff joints, particularly in the morning before you've got out of bed.

You can buy **'wheat bags' that are microwaveable** to soothe joint pain, or you could make your own, by filling an old sock with wheat or rice and herbs and tying the end up.

Use a **hot water bottle** on your joints in bed if they are cold or painful.

Therapeutic support gloves help to reduce pain and swelling in the hands and make them feel more comfortable.

Leisure

Gardening

When **planting seeds,** you may find it useful to use salt/pepper pots to sprinkle out small seeds that are difficult to pick up.

A border spade is lighter and easier to handle than a digging spade.

A stainless-steel blade is better than carbon steel as less soil clings to it making it easier to lift.

Spades with extra-long handles reduce the need to bend.

Weeding: You can reduce the number of weeds you have to deal with by covering the soil with a 5 cm (2-inch) layer of **shredded bark**. This excludes light from the soil and suppresses weed germination.

Pruning: A two-handed lopper will give you good leverage without much effort, protecting the finger joints from strain.

Other leisure tips

Computer mice or is it mouses?! Try out different types before choosing a suitable computer mouse. Some people find a rollerball is easier to use. The' Logitech' cordless trackman may be useful and wireless versions.

Use a Gimble **book holder** for hands free reading or lay the book on a table.

Use a **Kindle electronic reading device** then you do not need to hold the book or if you do it's very light.

Having a **pillow** with an integral speaker means you can listen to the radio at night without disturbing your partner! You could of course use headphones.

The Nintendo **Wii Fit and Wii fit plus** are great fun for exercise in your home.

Use a **dance exercise DVD** to allow you to exercise in the comfort of your own home at your own pace.

Dog walking: Use **a "Crufts" dog lead**. It has a padded handle. Useful if walking the dog on a less good day.

A-Z Guide to Wellbeing

A. Adapting and Accepting.

Adapting is key to achieving a good quality of life but also maintaining your health at an optimum level. It is about making changes so that you can still do many of the things that you want to. It is about finding new ways to achieve goals. It is about looking for alternatives that you can also enjoy.

A. Acceptance.

This is about accepting your illness or disability but NOT about giving up.

It is about accepting the position you find yourself in but moving forward.

B. Balance of Activities.

This is essential so that you do not put too much strain on any particular joint and so that you conserve energy for what is important to you.

Balance is also important when you have to trade off the benefits of medication against the side effects.

C. Choosing with Care.

Choosing correctly when you are buying new household equipment, tools or clothes is always essential. It can make the difference to being independent or dependant. It can also save the strain on your joints and prevent pain. Whether it's a new cooker, a new trowel or a new bed.

Try before you **Buy**

D. Disability Discrimination Act

As a person with a disability, you are entitled to access employment, public services and entertainment facilities. Whatever disability anyone has they should be treated with the same respect as anyone else. Employers and people selling goods and providing services will need to make reasonable adjustments for you.

E. Employment.

This is important whether your work is paid or voluntary. People gain self- respect and satisfaction from working as well as gaining benefits of socialising. They feel more confident and can maintain and update their skills. Work also gives us a sense of purpose and a feeling of being needed as well as giving a structure to the day.

F. Family and Friends.

Family and friends are essential for your wellbeing, social life, companionship and fun and you can help and support each other. They need to allow you to be independent but should also be able to give support when it is needed. They can be there as a listener, or they can give practical help.

G. Gratitude and Appreciation

Think about the things that you have enjoyed and appreciated every day. This might be seeing a friend, eating something that tasted wonderful, watching a great film, going for a walk or achieving a goal.

H. Heat.

The application of heat to joints is also a wonderful way of soothing away pain. Buy a heat pack or have a warm bath or shower. There are also tubs of wax that you can use to improve the circulation of the hands and thermal foot-spas too.

I. Independence.

This is about living your life and taking control of it. You do not have to be able to do everything for yourself to achieve independence. You can enlist some help as long as **you** make the decisions. Independence is very important for most people.

J. Joint Protection.

This is the way to maintain the joints as long as you can. There are three main concepts. These are avoidance of static positions, discouraging deformities and energy conservation techniques. Learn the basics and use them daily.

K. Keep moving.

This is a very important because it will help you to reduce stiffness and pain and will help you to maintain a good range of movements at the joints. It is important to use different joints by changing activities and positions.

L. Laughter.

Try and find something to have a good laugh at everyday. It could be spontaneous laughter with friends or colleagues, a comedy programme, jokes in books or on the internet. Remember laughter helps the feel-good endorphins to flow. Being able to laugh at yourself is useful too.

M. Medication.

Essential for controlling your disease but always know what you are taking and why and find out as much as you can about it.

Information is not always forthcoming, and you need to know the pros and cons of any medication that you take. Medication should be reviewed and blood tests carried out regularly if needed.

N. Nutritional intake.

It is important to eat well so that bones and muscles stay strong and that your general health is good. Try not to become overweight because all your joints will have to work so much harder to cope and so will your heart and lungs.

O. Optimism.

Remember optimists stay much healthier and generally live longer than pessimists. Whilst people who catastrophise generally have worse outcomes for their health. Try to look on the bright side whenever possible.

P. Positive Thinking.

This refers to making changes in the way you think about things. If you tend to view situations and events negatively then you need to look at alternative ways of interpreting them. This is called cognitive therapy. There are courses and books that can help you. Changing your thinking pattern takes time and practise.

Q. Questions.

Always arm yourself with information from books, from websites, from health practitioners and anyone who can offer a useful tip. It is only possible to take responsibility for your health and make informed decisions if you have knowledge so keep asking questions!

R. Relaxation and Rest.

These are both essential, but both are different.

Rest can be applied to any part of the body or all of it but the mind probably will not be included. It is certainly beneficial for the joints, but the mind can still be working hard.

Relaxation is about giving you a complete break from work or any ongoing problems and it certainly includes the mind. Relaxation is normally thought to include the relaxing of muscles, as in relaxation techniques but the relaxing of the mind as in meditation or visualization or guided fantasies is very important. I would also include absorbing the mind in an activity you enjoy even though the mind and body may still be active.

S. Specialised equipment and Splints.

There are many gadgets available to enable you to carry on doing what you want to do. Alternatively, you may well come up with your own ideas. Remember try before you buy whenever possible.

Splints

Work splints or nocturnal resting splints can be provided by the Occupational Therapy department and are useful to help you reduce your pain.

T. Taking Responsibility.

We have all become too dependent on expecting medical practitioners to give us a quick fix. We need to be involved in helping ourselves as much as possible with the support and guidance of the medical profession. Ideally there should be a partnership with both of us contributing in order to maintain good health. Consultants should be just that i.e. someone to consult with but the choices need to be made by the patient in conjunction with the practitioner.

U. Universal Credit and Disability Benefits.

These benefits can be important to allow you to be able to buy special equipment that you need or care that you require or it could be necessary to pay for an adapted car or a taxi fare or to reduce work hours when you are struggling. Having a disability always costs you extra money.

V. Vegetarianism.

Give this a try to see if the symptoms of RA subside. There is some evidence that it works for some people however we are all different and what works for one may not work for another.

W. Well-being.

This is the term for the way that you feel about yourself and your health. It has nothing to do with the medical conditions you may have. It is the way you feel about your own life and health that counts.

X. X Rays and Scans

Great for working out what is wrong. You can then work out a plan of action with your doctor or consultant.

Y. Yoga.

This is a very beneficial activity that will help you to keep the full range of movements in the joints, a supple body and strong muscles. It is also useful to relax the mind.

Z. Zingiber Officinale.

This is the Chinese name for ginger. It is thought to contain anti-inflammatory properties. It can be cooked and eaten in meals, or you can drink it in herbal teas or take it as a supplement.

Bibliography

Burnell, C; I Am Not A Label: 34 disabled artists, thinkers, athletes and activists from past and present (Quarto Publishing PLC, 2021)

Disability Rights UK; Disability Rights Handbook: 2023-2024 (Disability Rights UK, 2023)

Elton, K; A Resilient Life: Learning to thrive not just survive with rheumatoid arthritis (Kathryn Elton, 2010)

Firth, L; Living with Disability (Independence, *Educational Publishers*, 2010)

Fraser, H; The Little Big Things: A Young Man's Belief That Every Day Can Be a Good Day (Seven Dials, 2018)

Gupta, N; Rheumatoid Arthritis: A Doctor's Advice: Blueprint to Pain Free Life (Amazon, 2020)

Moyes, J; Me Before You (Penguin USA, 2012)

Taussig, R; Sitting Pretty: The View from My Ordinary Resilient Disabled Body (HarperCollins Publishers Inc, 2021)

Webster, L; The View from Down Here: Life as a Young Disabled Women (Dorling Kingsley Ltd, 2023)

Wong, A; Disability Visibility: First-Person Stories from the Twenty-First Century (Vintage, 2020)

Information publications

National Rheumatoid Arthritis Society: Living better with RA, Fatigue Matters, Blood Matters, I want to work (NRAS, 2024)

References

Chapter 3 The Second Decade; The Diagnosis

1 Foxton, P (2025) nras.org.uk

2 Rheumatoid Arthritis and Fatigue (2014) nras.org.uk/resource

Chapter 4 The Third Decade; Working Life

3 Definition of Disability under the Equality Act (2010) gov.uk/definition-of-disability-under-equality-act-2010

4 Webster, L (2023) The View from Down here (Dorling Kingsley Ltd)

Chapter 5 The Fourth Decade; Freedom to Travel

5 Official Statistics (2025) The Employment of Disabled People 2024 gov.uk/the employment of disabled people

6 The DAS 28 score (2025) nras.org/resource

Chapter 6 The Fifth Decade; Life After Work

7 The NHS Gym/Exercise Referral scheme (2025) the fitnessgrp.co.uk/nhs-gp-exercise-referral-scheme

8 MacPherson, Dr H *et al* (2017) Acupuncture is of benefit to some types of chronic pain york.ac.uk

9 Benefits of the Mediterranean anti-inflammatory diet, (2025) nras.org/resource/diet

10 Nutrition Interventions in Rheumatoid Arthritis: The Potential Use of Plant-Based Diets. A Review, (2019)

https://www.frontiersin.org/journals/nutrition/articles/10.3389/fnut.2019.00141/full

11 Rheumatoid Arthritis and Diet (2025) factsheet, bda.uk.com

12 Best foods for Rheumatoid Arthritis (2025) Arthritis Foundation arthritis.org

Chapter 7 Some Positive Changes for RA 1974-2024

13 Davis, P; (1998) Gold Therapy in the Treatment of Rheumatoid Arthritis Feb;34:445, 447, 449, 451- [452].

14 Rheumatoid arthritis in adults: management (2025) nice.org.uk/guidance

15 Rheumatoid Arthritis and Surgery (2025) nras/resource/surgery

16 Rheumatoid Arthritis and Surgery (2025) nras/resource/surgery

17 Louie G H, Ward M M, Changes in the rates of Joint Surgery among patients with Rheumatoid Arthritis in California, 1983-2007
https://www.ncbi.nlm.nih.gov/pmc/articles/PMC2859109/

18 Attitudinal Barriers,(2025)
https://www.inclusionlondon.org.uk/about-us/disability-in-london/social-model/the-social-model-of-disability

Chapter 8 Achieving a Positive Outlook

19 Parker, J *et al* (1988) *Journal of Rheumatology*, Sept; 15(9): 1376-83

20 Bentsen, P and Hornquist, JO (1994) *Scandinavian Journal of Social Medicine*, June;22(2):87-106

21 Keefe, F *et al* (1989) *Pain*, 37: 51-6

22 Riemsma, RP *et al* (1998) *British Journal of Rheumatology*, Oct; 37(10):1042-6

23 Hagglund, KJ *et al* (1989) *Arthritis and Rheumatism*, July; 32(7) ;851-8

24 Seligman, M (11998) Learned optimism, in Manning, M, *The Healing Journey*. Piatkus

25 Achat, H *et al* (2000) *Annals of Behavioural Medicine*, Spring; 22(2):127-30

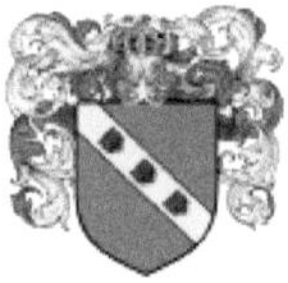

9781917525572

BV - #0054 - 011225 - C0 - 210/148/10 - PB - 9781917525572 - Gloss Lamination